Lassa Fever

Lassa Fever

Viral Replication, Disease Pathogenesis, and Host Immune Modulations

Editor

Hinh Ly

MDPI • Basel • Beijing • Wuhan • Barcelona • Belgrade • Manchester • Tokyo • Cluj • Tianjin

Editor
Hinh Ly
University of Minnesota
USA

Editorial Office
MDPI
St. Alban-Anlage 66
4052 Basel, Switzerland

This is a reprint of articles from the Special Issue published online in the open access journal *Pathogens* (ISSN 2076-0817) (available at: https://www.mdpi.com/journal/pathogens/special_issues/Lassa_Fever_Viral_Replication_Disease_Pathogenesis_Host_Immune_Modulations).

For citation purposes, cite each article independently as indicated on the article page online and as indicated below:

LastName, A.A.; LastName, B.B.; LastName, C.C. Article Title. *Journal Name* **Year**, *Article Number*, Page Range.

ISBN 978-3-03936-609-5 (Hbk)
ISBN 978-3-03936-610-1 (PDF)

Contents

About the Editor . . . . **vii**

Hinh Ly
Lassa Fever: Viral Replication, Disease Pathogenesis, and Host Immune Modulations
Reprinted from: *Pathogens* **2020**, *9*, 437, doi:10.3390/pathogens9060437 . . . . **1**

Rachel A. Sattler, Slobodan Paessler, Hinh Ly and Cheng Huang
Animal Models of Lassa Fever
Reprinted from: *Pathogens* **2020**, *9*, 197, doi:10.3390/pathogens9030197 . . . . **5**

María Eugenia Loureiro, Alejandra D'Antuono and Nora López
Virus–Host Interactions Involved in Lassa Virus Entry and Genome Replication
Reprinted from: *Pathogens* **2019**, *8*, 17, doi:10.3390/pathogens8010017 . . . . **27**

Katherine A. Willard, Jacob T. Alston, Marissa Acciani and Melinda A. Brindley
Identification of Residues in Lassa Virus Glycoprotein Subunit 2 That Are Critical for Protein Function
Reprinted from: *Pathogens* **2019**, *8*, 1, doi:10.3390/pathogens8010001 . . . . **45**

Christopher M. Ziegler, Philip Eisenhauer, Inessa Manuelyan, Marion E. Weir, Emily A. Bruce, Bryan A. Ballif and Jason Botten
Host-Driven Phosphorylation Appears to Regulate the Budding Activity of the Lassa Virus Matrix Protein
Reprinted from: *Pathogens* **2018**, *7*, 97, doi:10.3390/pathogens7040097 . . . . **59**

Juan Carlos Zapata, Sandra Medina-Moreno, Camila Guzmán-Cardozo and Maria S. Salvato
Improving the Breadth of the Host's Immune Response to Lassa Virus
Reprinted from: *Pathogens* **2018**, *7*, 84, doi:10.3390/pathogens7040084 . . . . **73**

Dylan M. Johnson, Jenny D. Jokinen and Igor S. Lukashevich
Attenuated Replication of Lassa Virus Vaccine Candidate ML29 in STAT-1$^{-/-}$ Mice
Reprinted from: *Pathogens* **2019**, *8*, 9, doi:10.3390/pathogens8010009 . . . . **91**

Maria S. Salvato, Arban Domi, Camila Guzmán-Cardozo, Sandra Medina-Moreno, Juan Carlos Zapata, Haoting Hsu, Nathanael McCurley, Rahul Basu, Mary Hauser, Michael Hellerstein and Farshad Guirakhoo
A Single Dose of Modified Vaccinia Ankara Expressing Lassa Virus-like Particles Protects Mice from Lethal Intra-cerebral Virus Challenge
Reprinted from: *Pathogens* **2019**, *8*, 133, doi:10.3390/pathogens8030133 . . . . **109**

About the Editor

Hinh Ly, Ph.D., Professor. Dr. Ly received his B.S. and M.A. degrees with honors in Microbiology and Molecular Genetics from the University of California, Los Angeles (UCLA), in 1995 and 1998, respectively, and his Ph.D. degree in Microbiology and Immunology from the University of North Carolina at Chapel Hill (UNC) in 2000. He completed a postdoctoral fellowship at the University of California, San Francisco (UCSF) in 2003. Prior to his current position as a Tenured and Full Professor in the Department of Veterinary Biomedical Sciences at the University of Minnesota, Twin Cities, Dr. Ly served as Assistant Professor in the Department of Pathology and Laboratory Medicine at Emory University in Atlanta. Dr. Ly's research interests have focused on virus-host interactions and vaccine and antiviral developments. Work in his laboratory has been consistently supported by the National Institutes of Health (NIH), the Department of Agriculture - National Institute of Food and Agriculture (USDA-NIFA), the Minnesota Agricultural Experiment Station, and other public, private and philanthropic organizations. He serves as a frequent reviewer of grant applications for the NIH, the Department of Defense (DoD) and other national and international agencies. He is currently serving as Director of Graduate Studies at the University of Minnesota and on the editorial board of several scientific journals, and is Section Editor of Virulence and Deputy Editor-in-Chief of the Journal of Medical Virology.

pathogens

MDPI

Editorial

Lassa Fever: Viral Replication, Disease Pathogenesis, and Host Immune Modulations

Hinh Ly

Department of Veterinary Biomedical Sciences, University of Minnesota, Twin Cities, 1988 Fitch Ave., Ste. 295, Saint Paul, MN 55108, USA; hly@umn.edu; Tel.: +612-625-3358; Fax: +612-625-0204

Received: 28 May 2020; Accepted: 2 June 2020; Published: 3 June 2020

Abstract: Despite major discoveries made in the last few decades about Lassa fever, there are still many unresolved key issues that hamper the development of effective vaccines and therapies against this deadly disease that is endemic in several West African countries. Some of these issues include the lack of a detailed understanding of the viral and participating host factors in completing the virus life cycle, in mediating disease pathogenesis or protection from disease, and in activating or suppressing host innate and cellular immunity against virus infection, as well as of the animal models required for testing vaccines and therapeutics. This Special Issue is devoted to understanding some of these important issues and to exploring the current status of the research and development in combating Lassa fever.

Keywords: Lassa virus; arenavirus; mammarenavirus; vaccine; virulence; pathogenesis; innate immunity; adaptive immunity; COVID-19

Since the first case of the new coronavirus disease in 2019 (COVID-19) was reported on 25 February 2020 in Algeria (North Africa), the overall numbers of reported cases and deaths have been increasing exponentially in recent weeks in Africa, with all 47 member states of the WHO African Region being affected, and more than half of the countries in the region are experiencing community transmission (https://www.afro.who.int/health-topics/coronavirus-covid-19). As of 19 May 2020, the highest case load has been observed in West African regions at 40% of the total number of cases (24,836 cases with a case fatality rate (CFR) of 2.2%), followed by the Southern African region at 27% (17,450, CFR 1.8%), the North African region at 8.5% (7377, CFR 7.6%), the Central African region at 15% (9331, CFR 3.2%), and the East African region at 7% (4506, CFR 2.4%). A major concern is that the current COVID-19 pandemic might become endemic in some countries in Africa and around the globe. It is important to note that other infectious diseases, such as HIV, malaria, and Lassa fever, have already been endemic for many decades in Africa, in particular in Sub-Saharan Africa. It is, therefore, important not to lose sight of these ongoing pandemic and endemic infections and the potential of the co-circulation of these deadly human pathogens in these regions where health care and social and political conditions (in some countries) are highly unstable.

In this Special Issue, that is devoted to understanding some of the important issues about Lassa fever that is endemic in several West African nations, there are seven timely contributions in the form of original research and review articles on Lassa fever's viral replication, the disease pathogenesis and protection, host immune modulations, and other related hot topics. In particular, three review articles contributed by leading researchers in the field that cover important concepts, including how different animal models can be developed for understanding Lassa fever's disease pathogenesis and pathologies and for the evaluation of candidate vaccines and antiviral therapies [1], how to improve the breadth of host immune responses to Lassa vaccination [2], as well as how different virus and host factors orchestrate the intricate processes of Lassa virus (LASV) entry and genome replication [3]. In addition to these insightful review articles, two research articles deal with novel strategies of developing vaccines for Lassa fever, including the use of the LASV-like particles composed of the viral matrix (Z) and envelope glycoprotein complex (GPC) expressed by the modified vaccinia Ankara virus to protect mice against lethal virus challenges [4] and the use of a candidate LASV vaccine known as ML29 that is composed of the reassorted genome between the pathogenic LASV and the non-pathogenic Mopeia virus (MOPV), which shows its highly attenuated phenotype in rodents [5]. An intriguing observation from this study is that the persistent infection of cells with ML29 can result in the generation of interfering viral particles that can induce a potent level of cell-mediated immunity and can strongly interfere with the replication of arenaviruses, such as LASV, MOPV, and lymphocytic choriomeningitis virus (LCMV).

There are two other research papers that cover some hot topics in the field. One such paper uses state-of-the-art mass spectrometry to identify novel phosphorylation sites in the LASV Z protein [6]. In particular, residues of two serines (S18, S98) and a tyrosine (Y97) located in the flexible N- and C-terminal regions of the protein are found be phosphorylated. Two of these residues, Y97 and S98, happen to be located in or directly adjacent to the so-called late domain with the PPXY motif, which is known to be required for mediating optimal progeny virion release from the infected cells. The authors showed that phosphorylation of these amino acids served as an important regulatory mechanism of virus release and that host-driven, reversible phosphorylation processes might play an important role in the regulation of LASV Z protein function in virus assembly and release.

Another important step in the life cycle of LASV is viral entry, which is a two-step process that involves the viral envelope glycoprotein complex (GPC). The GP subunit 1 (GP1) of the GPC first binds to the cell surface receptor before the viral particle is engulfed into the cellular endosome. A drop in pH in the endosome triggers GPC structural rearrangements which lead the GP subunit 2 (GP2) of the GPC to form a six-helix-bundle that helps fuse the lysosomal membrane with the LASV envelope membrane, allowing the LASV genome to enter the cellular cytoplasm for replication and transcription. In order to identify amino acid residues in GP2 that are crucial for the process of LASV entry, Willard and colleagues performed a semi-saturated alanine scanning mutagenesis of amino acid residues of GP2 [7]. They tested these mutant GPCs for efficient GP1-GP2 cleavage, cell-to-cell membrane fusion, and transduction into cells expressing the known cellular receptor (α-dystroglycan) and other secondary LASV receptors. Using this systematic experimental approach, the authors successfully identified seven GP2 mutants that could mediate efficient GP1-GP2 cleavage, yet they were unable to effectively transduce cells, which suggests that these key residues are critically important for GP2 function in the process of LASV entry into cells.

Funding: NIH NIAID (R01 AI131586), USDA NIFA (2019-05384), and the Minnesota Agricultural Experiment Station's Rapid Agriculture Response Fund (AES00RR245).

Acknowledgments: Work in the author's laboratory is supported by grants from the National Institutes of Health (NIH) National Institute of Allergy and Infectious Diseases (NIAID), US Department of Agriculture (USDA) National Institute of Food and Agriculture (NIFA), and the Minnesota Agricultural Experiment Station. The author would like to thank all authors of the contributing articles in this Special Issue for their insights, enthusiasm, and timely contributions.

Conflicts of Interest: The author declares no conflict of interest.

References

1. Sattler, R.; Paessler, S.; Ly, H.; Huang, C. Animal Models of Lassa Fever. *Pathogens* **2020**, *9*, 197. [CrossRef] [PubMed]
2. Zapata, J.C.; Medina-Moreno, S.M.; Guzmán-Cardozo, C.; Salvato, M.S. Improving the Breadth of the Host's Immune Response to Lassa Virus. *Pathogens* **2018**, *7*, 84. [CrossRef] [PubMed]
3. Loureiro, M.E.; D'Antuono, A.; López, N. Virus–Host Interactions Involved in Lassa Virus Entry and Genome Replication. *Pathogens* **2019**, *8*, 17. [CrossRef] [PubMed]
4. Salvato, M.S.; Domi, A.; Guzmán-Cardozo, C.; Medina-Moreno, S.; Zapata, J.C.; Hsu, H.; McCurley, N.; Basu, R.; Hauser, M.; Hellerstein, M.; et al. A Single Dose of Modified Vaccinia Ankara Expressing

Lassa Virus-like Particles Protects Mice from Lethal Intra-cerebral Virus Challenge. *Pathogens* **2019**, *8*, 133. [CrossRef]
5. Johnson, D.M.; Jokinen, J.D.; Lukashevich, I.S. Attenuated Replication of Lassa Virus Vaccine Candidate ML29 in STAT-1$^{-/-}$ Mice. *Pathogens* **2019**, *8*, 9. [CrossRef] [PubMed]
6. Ziegler, C.M.; Eisenhauer, P.; Manuelyan, I.; Weir, M.E.; Bruce, E.A.; Ballif, B.A.; Botten, J.W. Host-Driven Phosphorylation Appears to Regulate the Budding Activity of the Lassa Virus Matrix Protein. *Pathogens* **2018**, *7*, 97. [CrossRef] [PubMed]
7. Willard, K.A.; Alston, J.T.; Acciani, M.; Brindley, M.A. Identification of Residues in Lassa Virus Glycoprotein Subunit 2 That Are Critical for Protein Function. *Pathogens* **2018**, *8*, 1. [CrossRef] [PubMed]

pathogens

MDPI

Review

Animal Models of Lassa Fever

Rachel A. Sattler [1], Slobodan Paessler [1], Hinh Ly [2] and Cheng Huang [1,*]

[1] Department of Pathology, University of Texas Medical Branch, 301 University Blvd., Galveston, TX 77555-0609, USA; rasattle@utmb.edu (R.A.S.); slpaessl@utmb.edu (S.P.)

[2] Department of Veterinary Biomedical Sciences, University of Minnesota, Twin Cities, 1988 Fitch Ave., 295H Animal Science Veterinary Medicine Bldg., Saint Paul, MN 55108, USA; hly@umn.edu

* Correspondence: chhuang@utmb.edu; Tel.: +1-409-266-6934

Received: 27 January 2020; Accepted: 27 February 2020; Published: 6 March 2020

Abstract: Lassa virus (LASV), the causative agent of Lassa fever, is estimated to be responsible for up to 300,000 new infections and 5000 deaths each year across Western Africa. The most recent 2018 and 2019 Nigerian outbreaks featured alarmingly high fatality rates of up to 25.4%. In addition to the severity and high fatality of the disease, a significant population of survivors suffer from long-term sequelae, such as sensorineural hearing loss, resulting in a huge socioeconomic burden in endemic regions. There are no Food and Drug Administration (FDA)-approved vaccines, and therapeutics remain extremely limited for Lassa fever. Development of countermeasures depends on relevant animal models that can develop a disease strongly mimicking the pathogenic features of Lassa fever in humans. The objective of this review is to evaluate the currently available animal models for LASV infection with an emphasis on their pathogenic and histologic characteristics as well as recent advances in the development of a suitable rodent model. This information may facilitate the development of an improved animal model for understanding disease pathogenesis of Lassa fever and for vaccine or antiviral testing.

Keywords: arenaviruses; Lassa virus; viral hemorrhagic fevers; Lassa fever; animal models

---

1. Introduction

Lassa virus (LASV) is the causative agent of Lassa fever (LF). The virus was first isolated from two missionary nurses who died from LF in Nigeria in 1969 [1–3]. A third nurse was infected and brought to the United States; her plasma was used to treat a fourth patient who was exposed by handling infected blood samples [1]. LASV is a mammarenavirus from the *Arenaviridae* family and has a single-stranded, negative-sense, bisegmented RNA genome. LASV is endemic throughout Western Africa, especially in Nigeria, Liberia, Guinea, and Sierra Leone, where it is transmitted by the Natal mastomys (*Mastomys natalensis*) rodent, although recent work suggests viral presence in the reddish-white mastomys (*Mastomys erythroleucus*) and the "African wood mouse" (*Hylomyscus pamfi*) rodents as well [2,4]. LASV isolates of different geographic and host origins are highly diverse in genomic sequences and phylogenetically classified into up to seven lineages, with each lineage predominately localized in specific countries (refer to Table 1 for the LASV isolates covered in this review) [5–9]. A recent deep sequencing analysis revealed that the sequence variations could be as high as 25% and 32% in the viral genomic small (S) and large (L) segments, respectively, among different strains [5]. LASV causes zoonotic infections in humans, typically through the ingestion of contaminated food and/or water or inhalation of tainted aerosols from infected rodents; person-to-person transmission occurs via contact with bodily fluids [2]. Estimates from the Centers for Disease Control and Prevention (CDC) place the number of new LASV infections each year as high as 300,000 with around 5000 deaths from LF [2,10]. The average case fatality rate is approximately 1%, which can dramatically elevate to 15–20% for hospitalized cases [2]. However, a more recent report indicated only 633 confirmed cases and 171 deaths in Nigeria in 2018, with a 27% case fatality rate [11]. In the recent 2018–2019 Nigerian LF outbreaks, approximately 25% of patients died from the infection [12–14]. Therefore, it is necessary to re-evaluate the annual incidence of LASV infections and deaths.

There are no FDA-approved vaccines against LASV. Current clinical treatments are limited to an off-label use of ribavirin [2,14]. However, ribavirin treatment is expensive and only effective if administered within the first six days after the onset of symptoms [15]. When considering the high rate of misdiagnosis of LF for other endemic infections, such as typhoid or falciparum malaria [1,2,16,17], this time frame for effective LF treatment is extremely challenging [16]. Moreover, ribavirin has a high rate of side effects that often require further medical intervention, such as hemolysis [15]. Development of countermeasures against LF requires relevant animal models that can recapitulate disease and pathogenic features of LF in humans. The objective of this review is to survey the current Lassa fever animal models, including their pathologic and histologic characteristics as well as new advances in small rodent models, in order to inform the development of new animal models.

Table 1. Information for Lassa virus (LASV) strains examined in animal models *.

Strain	Lineage	Lethal/Fatal	Host	Isolation Country	Isolation Year	Reference
Josiah	IV	Yes	Human	Sierra Leone	1976	[6]
AV	V	Yes	Human	Ghana/Ivory Coast	2000	[6]
Ba366	IV	No	*Mastomys natalensis*	Guinea	2003	[6]
LF2384	IV	Yes	Human	Sierra Leone	2012	[6,8]
LF2450	IV	No	Human	Sierra Leone	2012	[6,8]
Soromba-R	V	No	*Mastomys natalensis*	Soromba, Mali	2009	[6]
Pinneo	I	No	Human	Lassa, Nigeria	1969	[6]
NJ2015	IV	Yes	Human	Liberia	2015	[9]

* Only strains mentioned in this review that have known isolation information are listed in this table.

2. Lassa Fever Symptoms and Pathogenesis

LF symptoms typically appear 1–3 weeks post-infection [2]. Eighty percent of cases are asymptomatic or present with mild, non-specific febrile symptoms such as fever, sore throat, headache, and general malaise, that may be misdiagnosed as typhoid, malaria, or appendicitis [1,2,16,17]. The other 20% of cases progress to much more severe symptomology [2]. These clinical manifestations include diarrhea, hemorrhage, disorientation, respiratory distress, abdominal pain, vomiting, facial edema, and severe pharyngitis [1,2]. Neurological signs such as hearing loss, encephalitis, and tremors also occur [2]. Of note, this hearing loss manifests as sudden-onset sensorineural hearing loss (SNHL) in approximately one-third of patients and is irreversible in two-thirds of those cases [10,18,19]. Infections during pregnancy have a greater risk of death as well as spontaneous abortion [20]. Death will typically occur due to multiorgan failure approximately two weeks post-onset of symptoms [2]. The long-term sequelae, such as SNHL, are generating a huge socioeconomic burden across Western Africa, where stigmatization and isolation lead to increased rates of depression and unemployment [21]. Aid programs in Nigeria alone can cost upwards of $43 million each year [18].

Clinical laboratory findings include thrombocytopenia, leucopenia with lymphopenia, elevated blood urea and proteinuria [22]. The aspartate aminotransferase (AST), alanine aminotransferase (ALT), amylase, and creatine phosphokinase (CPK) concentrations are also elevated in patient's serum [17], often with a higher AST level than ALT level, suggesting that the transaminases in serum are not solely derived from damaged liver, but may also be from other tissues [23]. High viral titers are measured in the spleen, lung, liver, kidney, heart, mammary gland, and placenta [17]. The level of viremia has been correlated with the severity of disease outcome.

Current knowledge on the pathology of Lassa fever is still limited due to civil unrest and social taboos and customs when dealing with the deceased in endemic areas [22]. Available pathologic analysis of clinical cases indicates lesions in the spleen, liver, and adrenal glands [17]. Histologic analysis of the liver indicates significant eosinophilic necrosis and parenchymal cell necrosis with an infiltration of eosinophils in the sinusoids [1,17,24]. Spleen samples indicate a presence of eosinophilic necrosis, lymphoid depletion, atrophied white pulp, and fibrin deposits with an infiltration of lymphocytes and mononuclear cells [1,17,24]. Adrenal gland samples indicate multifocal adrenocortical cellular necrosis, often associated with inflammation [17]. Less frequent findings include petechiae of the gastrointestinal tract, interstitial nephritis, renal tubular injury, lymph node sinus histiocytosis, mild interstitial pneumonia, renal edema and hemorrhage, as well as mild interstitial mononuclear myocarditis [1,17,24]. No alterations are detected in placental, mammary, uterine, ovarian, pancreatic, central nervous system (CNS), or brain samples [17]. These observations were made from a study performed in 1982. Our knowledge on pathology of LF in humans still lack. Studies with non-human primates have provided valuable information regarding the pathogenesis of LASV infection. As there is a limitation in study with non-human primates (NHPs), a small animal model that can resemble pathological changes in LF patients is desired.

3. Murine Models

3.1. Natal Mastomys (*Mastomys Natalensis*) Mice

Natal mastomys mice are the natural host of LASV. The exact subspecies that acts as a LASV reservoir remains unclear, due to multiple subspecies coexisting in endemic regions and their high genetic diversity [25,26]. There are very few studies on laboratory infections of Natal mastomys due to lack of laboratory clone of these mice. One early study reported that LASV caused a chronic asymptomatic infection despite the high virus titers detected in organs at 74 days post-infection (dpi) [25] (Table 2). Affected tissues included the lung, spleen, liver, kidney, brain, bladder, and lymph nodes [25]. Virus was also detected in the blood and urine. As the Natal mastomys mice did not develop LF signs, its use in viral pathogenesis or vaccine studies is limited. However, this model may prove useful for basic transmission studies as well as studies developing methods for limiting transmission of the virus between rodent populations or from rodents to humans.

Table 2. Mouse models of LASV infection.

Mouse	Virus Strain	Max. Dose	Route	Lethality	Signs of Disease	Affected Organs	Reference
Natal mastomys	Unknown	Not provided	IP [d]	No	asymptomatic, persistent infection, virus shed in saliva and urine	lung, spleen, liver, kidney, brain, bladder, lymph nodes	[25]
IFNAR$^{-/-}$	Josiah, AV, BA366, Nig04-10	10^5 PFU	IV [e]	No	persistent viremia, bodyweight loss, no fever and neurological signs	lung, liver, spleen brain, kidney, heart	[27–30]
Chimeric IFNAR$^{-/-B6}$	Ba366, AV, Ba289, Nig04-10, Nig-CSF	10^3 FFU	IP	100%	liver damage, vascular leakage, systemic viral dissemination, weight loss, hypothermia, elevated AST/ALT ratio	liver, lung, spleen, kidney, heart, brain	[29,31]
IFN$\alpha\beta/\gamma$R$^{-/-}$	Josiah, LF2384 [a] LF2450 [b]	10^5 PFU	IP	No	minor and transient weight loss, clearance of virus by 25 dpi, no hearing loss	spleen, lung, liver, brain, kidney	[8,30]
STAT1$^{-/-}$	Josiah	10^4 PFU	IP	100%	weight loss, systematic infection	spleen, lung, liver, brain, kidney	[28]
	LF2384 [a] (fatal)	10^5 PFU	IP	80%	fever, high level viremia, weight loss, increased ALT level, decreased albumin, WBC, and monocyte counts, hearing loss associated with infiltration of CD3$^+$ lymphocytes	brain, liver, spleen, lung, kidney, heart	[8,28]
	LF2450 [b] (non-fatal)	10^5 PFU	IP	0–50%	hearing loss	brain, liver, spleen, lung, kidney, heart	[8]
CBA	Josiah	10^3 PFU	IC [f]	70–100%	scruffy fur, seizures, weight loss, immobility, and severe decubitus paralysis	not stated	[32]
HHD	Ba366 [C]	10^6 PFU	IV	22%	ruffled fur, lethargy, elevated AST level, high level viremia, severe pneumonitis	liver, lung, spleen, kidney	[33]

Note: [a] LF2384: clinical isolate from a lethally infected patient; [b] LF2450: clinical isolate from a survivor; [C] isolate from *Natal mastomys*; PFU, plaque forming unit; [d] IP: intraperitoneal; [e] IV: intravenous; [f] IC: intracranial.

3.2. IFNAR$^{-/-}$ Mice

Immune-competent laboratory mice are generally resistant to LASV infection [27–30]. Interferons play important roles in regulating host innate and adaptive immune responses against infections. LASV infection of the 129Sv mice lacking the receptor for interferon α and β (IFNAR$^{-/-}$) results in a non-lethal acute infection accompanied with persistent viremia [27–30] (Table 2). Infected mice lose approximately 15% body weight but did not develop febrile or neurological signs [26,29]. Other disease signs included ruffled fur and hypoactivity occurring by 11 dpi [28,30]. Peak viremia occurred approximately 8 dpi. The lung, liver, and spleen had the highest viral loads, and virus was also present in the brain, kidney, and heart at much lower titers [27]. Similar pathological changes and disease signs were found in the animals upon infection with a variety of LASV strains, including the Josiah, AV, BA366, and Nig04-10 strains isolated from endemic countries, Sierra Leone, Côte d'Ivoire, Guinea, and Nigeria, respectively [27,28].

A chimeric IFNAR$^{-/-B6}$ lethal mouse model had been established, in which the IFNAR$^{-/-}$ mice were irradiated and transplanted with bone marrow progenitor cells from wild type C57BL/6 mice. These IFNAR$^{-/-B6}$ chimeric mice uniformly succumbed to infections with a variety of LASV strains within 10 days [29,31]. LASV strains tested include Ba366, AV, Ba289, Nig04-10, and Nig-CSF, all of which were 100% lethal using 1000 focus-forming units (FFU) [29]. These mice presented with liver damage, vascular leakage, and systemic viral dissemination [29]. Virus titers were detected in the liver, lung, spleen, kidney, heart, brain, and blood [29,31]. Animals also presented with weight loss and hypothermia [31]. Moreover, this model featured an elevated AST/ALT ratio, as well as FAS and FAS-L [29,31] similarly observed in LF patients. Pathological findings included an infiltration of inflammatory leukocytes in the kidney, infiltration of granulocytes and T cell lymphocytes in the liver, and an increased presence of CD8+ T cells in both the spleen and lungs [29]. Lung and liver samples both presented with indications of significant vascular leakage as well as edema [29]. Interestingly, IFNAR$^{-/-B6}$ mice with a depletion of CD8+ T cells exhibited significantly increased survival rate (87.5%) despite persistent viremia [29]. This depletion also reduced the FAS and FAS-L concentrations, as well as the vascular leakage in the liver and lung [29]. This model implicates the role of T cells in the pathogenesis of LF. IFNAR$^{-/-}$ mice are less susceptible to disease probably as a result of lacking IFN receptors that are critical to stimulate a T cell response.

3.3. *IFNαβ/γR$^{-/-}$ Mice*

The 129Sv mice lacking interferon α, β and γ receptors (IFNαβ/γR$^{-/-}$) did not develop clinical signs of disease upon LASV infection apart from a minor and transient weight loss [30] (Table 2). Neither did this model develop sudden onset sensorineural hearing loss when infected with either the LF2384 or LF2350 clinical isolates from a fatal and a non-fatal case respectively, from the 2012 Sierra Leone outbreak [8]. These two clinical isolates have been passaged only once in Vero cells. The animals presented with less severe disease upon infection with the Josiah strain as IFNAR$^{-/-}$ mice [30]. Virus was present in the serum, spleen, lung, liver, brain, and kidney, but was cleared by 25 dpi [30]. Tissue samples featured similar findings to the LASV-infected IFNAR$^{-/-}$ model in the brain and lung, but to significantly lesser extents [30]. Liver samples presented with mononuclear cell infiltration, although inflammation was rarely observed [30]. In the spleen, only the red pulp was affected; the kidneys showed mild, regional nephritis [30].

3.4. *STAT1$^{-/-}$ Mice*

Signal transducer and activator of transcription 1 (STAT1) is a transcription factor that is activated in response to IFN α, β, γ and IL-6. The 129Sv mice lacking STAT1 (STAT1$^{-/-}$) were not only highly susceptible to LASV infection, including clinical isolates, but also presented with a lethal disease with clinically relevant manifestations, such as SNHL [8,28]. Thus, the STAT1$^{-/-}$ mouse model is promising for vaccine and therapeutic testing. Mice intraperitoneally infected with 10^4 plaque forming units (PFUs) of the Josiah strain of LASV lost ~18% of their body weight between 4 and 6 dpi, and either died or met humane endpoint criteria by 7 dpi [28]. This model also matched the differential clinical outcome of the patients from whom the viruses were isolated, with LF2384 infections being lethal and LF2350 infections non-lethal in these mice. Intraperitoneal (IP) injection with 10^5 PFU of the LF2384 or the LF2350 isolates led to 80% and 10–50% lethality, respectively [8]. Infection with 10^4 PFU of these viruses resulted in 80% lethality for the fatal isolate and 0% lethality for the non-fatal isolate [8]. LF2384 also caused fever and other signs of disease by 4–5 dpi, and death approximately 7 dpi [28]. Other signs of disease included weight loss, hypothermia, hunched posture, reduced activity, and ruffled fur [8]. In one study, fever was not noted, although the possibility that fever transiently occurred before turning into hypothermia was raised [8,28]. Virus was disseminated to the brain, liver, spleen, lung, kidney, and heart by 3 dpi with titers steadily increasing to their peak at 7 dpi [8,28]. Viremia appeared by 3 dpi and remained at high titers until death [28]. Increased ALT concentrations and decreased albumin, WBC, and monocyte counts were noted as early as 3 dpi; a moderate decrease in platelet counts was also observed [28]. Histologic analysis of the spleen indicated lesions with eosinophil accumulation in the red pulp, primarily focused around the periarteriolar lymphocytic sheaths as well as apoptotic and necrotic cells [28]. Samples also demonstrated significant fibrin deposits and an infiltration of macrophages filled with apoptotic nuclei [28]. Analysis of the liver indicated lesions with microvesicular steatosis and apoptosis in the hepatic sinusoids [28]. Of note, IFN signaling is not completely disrupted in this STAT1$^{-/-}$ mouse model as that in IFN$\alpha\beta/\gamma R^{-/-}$ mice. A partial knockout of STAT1 gene leads to expression of a truncated form of STAT1, which may still be able to mediate a minimal T cell response. As T cells may contribute to LF pathogenesis, the difference in IFN signaling may explain why the STAT1$^{-/-}$ mice are more susceptible to disease than IFN$\alpha\beta/\gamma R^{-/-}$ mice [29].

Additionally, the STAT1$^{-/-}$ model is the only available small animal model for SNHL [8]. Both LF2384 and LF2350 clinical isolates from the 2012 Sierra Leone outbreak caused deafness in survivors [8]. Infection with 10^5 PFU of virus caused permanent hearing loss in all survivors. With a lower dose of virus (10^4 PFU), hearing loss was present in only 20% of survivors. Histologic examination identified severe damage to the inner ear with significantly fewer outer hair cells; inner hair cells remained intact [8]. Auditory nerves in mice with hearing loss were also damaged, while the nearby facial nerves remained intact. There was significant vacuolization of the spiral ganglion, thinning of the stria vascularis, distention of Reissner's membrane, and an infiltration of blood cells in the scala tympani. Viral antigen was present in vascular-rich regions, where there was also a remarkable infiltration of CD3+ lymphocytes, indicating an immunopathologic mechanism underlying to the hearing loss [8].

3.5. CBA Mice

Intracranial infection of inbred CBA mice with the pathogenic Josiah strain of LASV resulted in disease manifestation, although it was unclear whether the animals were immunocompromised [32]. Infected CBA mice presented with scruffy fur, seizures, weight loss, immobility, severe decubitus paralysis, and death [32]. This route of inoculation allowed for onset of signs of disease between 5 and 7 dpi with 70–100% lethality within 7–12 days [32].

3.6. HHD Mice

C57BL/6 mice expressing a human/mouse chimeric HLA-A2.1 instead of the normal MHC class I gene products (humanized HHD mouse model) has recently been established as a novel model for LASV infection [33]. The HHD mouse was most susceptible to infection with the Ba366 strain and featured ~22% lethality and rapid deteriorating post-onset of signs of disease [33]. When infected with 10^6 PFU of the Ba366 strain, HHD mice began to show ruffled fur and lethargy, as well as elevated concentrations of serum AST, approximately 7–12 dpi [33]. High viral titers were observed in liver, lung, and spleen, whereas lower titers were seen in the kidney [33]. Histology examination indicated severe pneumonitis with signs of pleural effusion, thickening of the interlobular septum, and collapsed alveolar lumen with infiltration of monocytes and macrophages [33]. The liver contained altered cellular distribution, orientation, and shape of its monocytes and macrophages. The spleens also featured disruption of the white and red pulp regions, while monocytes and macrophages were found throughout with scarce T cells.

Depletion of CD4+ T cells, CD8+ T cells, or both resulted in substantial differences in disease manifestations in this model [33]. After infection, the serum AST concentrations remained normal in HHD mice lacking both CD4+ and CD8+ T cells, while the AST concentrations elevated in HHD mice. Additionally, depletion of either CD4+ T cells or CD8+ T cells resulted in partial elevation in AST concentrations [33]. In all groups, similarly high titers of viremia were developed, suggesting T cells had no substantial influence on viremia. C57BL6 mice lacking only CD4+ T cells were able to clear the viral infection, while those lacking only the CD8+ cells featured persistent viremia [33]. MHC-I$^{-/-}$ mice lacking CD8+ T cells confirmed these findings, presenting with no clinical manifestations of disease after infection, despite the high viremia [33]. CD4+ and CD8+ T cell-depleted mice did not demonstrate any significant histological changes in the lung and spleen after infection and also featured limited signs of disease, emphasizing the role of T cells in LASV pathogenesis [33].

In summary, immune-competent laboratory mice are generally resistant to LASV infection, and therefore are not suitable for modeling the severe and fatal LF diseases in humans. Immune-incompetent mice are susceptible to LASV infection but generally develop mild diseases and survive the infection (see Table 2). The chimeric IFNAR$^{-/-B6}$ mice are susceptible to lethal LASV infection but require irradiation of the mice and transplantation with bone marrow progenitor cells from wild type C57BL/6 mice. Recently, progress has been made using the STAT1$^{-/-}$ mice, which recapitulate the pathogenic potency of different LASV isolates and some LF disease signs including hearing loss. This STAT1$^{-/-}$ mouse model may be useful as a small rodent model for vaccine and therapeutic testing.

4. Guinea Pig Models

4.1. Strain 13 Guinea Pigs

Inbred Strain 13 domesticated guinea pigs have been used as a lethal LF rodent model for studying pathogenesis as well as antiviral, vaccine, and immunotherapy candidates. Unlike their Hartley outbred counterpart, this model does not require virus adaptation [34,35] (Table 3). However, Inbred Strain 13 guinea pigs are not readily available, limiting their use as a LF animal model. In this model at least 90% animals died when infected with at least 2 PFU of LASV (Josiah) [34,36,37]. The clinical isolate NJ2015, from a non-fatal infection, was also non-lethal in Strain 13 guinea pigs [36]. Guinea pigs infected with the Pinneo strain had a 100% survival rate, developing only a mild to moderate disease featuring 5–10% weight loss and lethargy approximately 10 dpi; all animals recovered by 22 dpi [38]. The Z-132 strain was 100% lethal and mimicked a Josiah infection, while the Soromba-R strain was 0–57% lethal with a very mild disease [38,39]. Survivors did not exhibit seroconversion and were susceptible to back challenge [34]. Neutralizing antibodies were not produced [37]. Signs of disease included weight loss, fever, ruffled fur, hunched posture, altered mentation, and conjunctivitis [34–36]. Guinea pigs typically became moribund between 10 and 15 dpi [37]. A persistent and high level viremia developed rapidly, typically approximately 5–6 dpi, and peaked at approximately 10 dpi. The highest viral load was identified in the lung, followed by the spleen, pancreas, lymph nodes, adrenal glands, kidneys, salivary glands, liver, and heart [34,35,39]. Histological findings included the presence of viral antigen typically associated with hepatitis, hepatic cell death, hair follicle epithelium cell death, and adrenal cortical necrosis [35]. Laryngitis and heterophilic tracheitis were noted in guinea pigs exposed via aerosol [35]. Interstitial pneumonia was found in all moribund animals with an increase in mononuclear cells, especially macrophages, surrounding the blood vessels and airways [34,35,37,39]. Edema and hemorrhage were also noted in the lungs with an expansion of the alveolar septae [35,39]. Liver samples exhibited a mild to moderate inflammation in portal and sinusoidal regions, vacuolar degeneration, and necrosis [35,37,39]. Half of the guinea pigs developed acute necrotizing nephritis and mild myocarditis or mild to moderate endocarditis and pancarditis [34,35,37]. It is important to note that this damage to the heart is not seen in clinical cases [25]. Adrenal glands featured minimal damage, although they were infected [34,35]. Further analysis of the spleen identified mild heterophilic splenitis [35,39]. The red pulp featured perifollicular to diffuse mononuclear cell proliferation [35]. Most infected guinea pigs developed petechial rashes approximately 12 dpi [35]. Lymphocytolysis and lymphoid depletion was noted in the white pulp of the spleen, thymus, and lymph nodes [35,37]. The pancreas featured acinar cell atrophy as well as other architectural changes [35]. Viral antigen was present in the reproductive tissues of both male and female infected guinea pigs, with males also featuring mild epididymitis [35]. Serum analysis indicated elevated ALT and heterophil concentrations with a transient decrease in platelets and a decrease in blood lymphocytes [35].

Table 3. Guinea pig models of LASV infection.

Guinea Pig	Strain	Max. Dose	Route	Lethality	Signs of Disease	Affected Organs	Refences
Strain 13 (inbred)	Josiah	> 2 PFU10^4 $TCID_{50}$	SC [c] IP	>90%	weight loss, fever, ruffled fur, hunched posture, conjunctivitis, hepatitis, interstitial pneumonia, edema and hemorrhage in lungs	lung, spleen, pancreas, lymph nodes, adrenal and salivary glands, kidneys, liver, heart	[34,36,37]
	Z-132	10^4 $TCID_{50}$	IP	100%	Josiah-like	lung, liver, spleen	[38,39]
	Soromba-R	10^4 $TCID_{50}$	IP	0–57%	survivors only show minor weight loss	liver, lung, spleen	[28,34,35,38,39]
	Pinneo	10^4 $TCID_{50}$	IP	No	mild to moderate disease	N.A. *	[38]
	NJ2015	10^4 FFU	SC	No	weight loss, fever, red and swollen conjunctiva	eye (focus of the study)	[36]
Hartley (outbred)	Josiah	>2 PFU10^3 PFU	SCIP	30–67%	inapparent infection in survivors	N.A. *	[25,34,35,40,41]
	GPA-Josiah [a]	10^3 $TCID_{50}$	IP	100%	weight loss, fever, lethargy, respiratory distress, hypothermia	spleen, liver, lung	[25,34,35,40–42]
	LF2384 [b]	10^4 PFU	IP	100%	fever, weight loss, hypothermia, lethargy, thrombocytopenia, neutropenia, and lymphopenia	liver, kidney, spleen, lung, brain	[43]

* N.A: not available; [a] GPA-Josiah: guinea pig-adapted LASV Josiah strain; [b] LF2384: clinical isolate from a fatally infected LF patient; [c] SC: subcutaneous

Strain 13 guinea pigs presented with conjunctivitis upon LASV infection [36]. Clinically, LASV infections cause conjunctival edema and conjunctivitis in acute infections and transient blindness in survivors. No other animal models have been extensively studied for this aspect of disease, although viral titers have been identified in the aqueous humor of the eye of infected rhesus monkeys [36,44]. The lethal Josiah strain and the non-lethal NJ2015 clinical isolate both induced red and swollen conjunctiva with associated ocular discharge in the animals [36]. Viral antigen was detected in the eyes of all infected guinea pigs achieving humane euthanasia criteria, while none was detected in those of survivors [36]. Survivors presented with minimal to mild lymphocytic inflammation; lethal infections all presented with mild to moderate inflammation [36].

4.2. Hartley Guinea Pigs

Outbred Hartley domesticated guinea pigs are commercially available and susceptible to infection with the widely used Josiah strain of LASV (Table 3). However, the Josiah strain caused lethal infection in only 30–67% of animals regardless of the infection dose. Survivors seroconverted and were not susceptible to back challenge [34]. To achieve uniform lethality, the Josiah strain must be adapted in guinea pigs through serial passage [25,34,35,40,41]. Guinea pigs infected with the guinea pig-adapted LASV (GPA-LASV) developed a fever approximately 6–9 dpi as well as respiratory distress and hypothermia [41,42]. Weight loss was rapid and variable, ranging from 8% to over 20%, which is typical humane euthanasia criteria [40–42]. Other clinical manifestations included an unstable gait, a noticeable lack of grooming with associated rough/ruffled fur, delayed responsiveness/lethargy, recumbency, and a reddening of the footpads and ears [40,41]. Death occurred by an average of 15 dpi [41]. Viral titers were observed in the serum, spleen, liver, and lung [41,42]. Histologic analysis of the liver indicated lymphohistiocytic hepatitis and hepatocellular degeneration [41]. Spleen samples contained sinus histiocytosis and lung samples featured interstitial pneumonia [41]. The GPA-LASV/Hartley guinea pig model has been often used in development of antivirals and vaccine against LF [40–42].

Recently, new advances have been made in the development of the outbred LASV-infected Hartley guinea pig model by using the LF2384 clinical isolate. Uniform lethality could be achieved in outbred Hartley guinea pigs infected by the LF2384 clinical isolate without species-specific adaptation, at a dose as low as 100 PFU [45]. LF2384-infected guinea pigs presented with signs of disease such as fever, hypothermia before death, as well as weight loss by 10 dpi, scruffy coats by 12 dpi, and loss of appetite as well as lethargy by 13 dpi [45]. Neurological disease signs were not observed in this model [45]. Viral loads were detected in the liver, kidney, spleen, lung, and brain, but were not detectable in survivors of a low dose infection [45]. Guinea pigs succumbing to disease presented with thrombocytopenia, neutropenia, and lymphopenia [45]. Gross pathology indicated small spleens [45]. While this model requires further characterization, the advantages of this new LF model include the use of clinical isolates directly from patients without adaptation and the commercial availability of the animals. Additionally, the outbred background may allow for mimicking infections in humans with diverse genetic backgrounds. The newly developed LF2384 LASV/Hartley guinea pig model will be useful for vaccine and therapeutic development, which is demonstrated in a recent study showing that immunization with an adenovector-based LASV vaccine candidate efficaciously protected animals from lethal LASV infection [43].

5. Non-Human Primate Models

5.1. Squirrel Monkey Model

Squirrel monkeys (*Saimiri sciureus*) infected with the Bah strain of LASV developed variable disease. One out of four animals became moribund [46] (Table 4). These primates develop depression, tremors, drooling, anorexia, lassitude, and polydipsia as signs of disease. Serologic analysis indicated persistent viremia with no antibody development at 28 dpi [46]. High viral titers were detected primarily in the liver, kidney, and lymph nodes, while lower virus loads were found in the spleen, brain, liver, kidneys, adrenal gland, urine and heart [25,46]. The presence of the virus was associated with significant tissue necrosis [25]. Spleen and lymph node samples featured necrosis in the germinal centers; spleen samples and adrenal glands also contain regions of focal hemorrhage [46]. While the liver suffered from hepatitis with fatty metamorphosis and an infiltration of leukocytes and mononuclear cells, hepatocytic regeneration was noted [46]. Renal tubular necrosis and regeneration was present in the kidney, while heart samples featured severe myocarditis with vacuolar degeneration and necrosis [46]. Some animals developed neuropathology with chronic inflammation of the meninges, a significant infiltration of mononuclear cells and lymphocytes into the pancreas with acute arteritis, or minor pathologic changes in the adrenal gland, prostate, and bone marrow [46].

Table 4. Non-human primate (NHP) models of LASV infection [a].

NHP	LASV Strain	Max. Dose	Route	Lethality	Signs of Disease	Affected Organs	Reference
squirrel monkeys	Bah	$10^{6.8}$ $TCID_{50}$	IM [b]	25%	depression, tremors, drooling, anorexia, lassitude, polydipsia	liver, kidney, lymph nodes, spleen, brain, adrenal gland, heart	[46]
marmoset	Josiah	10^6 PFU	SC	100%	low fever, rapid weight loss, depression, anorexia, elevated concentrations of AST, ALT, alkaline phosphatase, decreased concentrations of albumin and platelet	liver, spleen, lymph nodes, kidney, lung, adrenal gland	[47]
rhesus monkey	Josiah	$10^{6.1}$ PFU	SC	50–60%	severe petechial rash, hiccups, lethargy, aphagia, huddled posture, constipation, conjunctivitis, anorexia, weight loss, decreased water intake/dehydration, facial and periorbital edema, bleeding from the gums and nares, cough, fever	adrenal glands, liver, lung, pancreas, brain, bone marrow, kidney, lymph nodes, spleen, muscle, heart, thymus, testis, salivary gland, CSF, intestines	[44,48,49]
"crab-eating" cynomolgus macaques	Josiah	10^4 PFU	IM	Up to 100%	fever, weight loss, lethargy, dull appearance, reluctance to move/hypoactivity, anorexia, rashes, facial edema, hunched posture, ruffled fur, piloerection, bleeding from puncture sites, dehydration, epistaxis, acute respiratory syndrome, neurological signs including deafness	lymph nodes, spleen, liver, reproductive organs, kidney, lung, heart, CNS	[38,39,50–53]
	Z-132	10^4 $TCID_{50}$	IM	100%	Josiah-like	spleen, liver, lung	[38,39]
	Soromba-R	10^4 $TCID_{50}$	IM	66%	less severe than Josiah strain infection, moderate to severe pulmonary lesions	similar to Josiah and Z-132	[39]

[a] Another NHP model, for which the literature was not available to the authors, is the hydramas baboon model; [b] IM: intramuscular.

5.2. Marmoset Model

The common marmoset (*Callithrix jacchus*) has been identified as a good model for Lassa fever (Table 4). Primates infected with the Josiah strain of LASV develop a systemic disease featuring low fever and rapid weight loss [47]. These monkeys also exhibited behavioral changes, such as depression and anorexia, as well as reduced stool production [47]. Severe morbidity occurred between 15 and 20 dpi [47]. Serum analysis indicated an elevation in AST, ALT, and alkaline phosphatase concentrations as well as a decrease in albumin and platelet concentrations [47]. High viral titers were observed in the liver, spleen, and lymph nodes [47]. Livers were enlarged with pale patches. Histologic analysis indicated multifocal hepatic necrosis with mild inflammation [47]. Spleens were also enlarged with mild to moderate lymphoid depletion [47]. Likewise, lymph nodes were enlarged with lymphocyte necrosis and an infiltration of inflammatory cells [47]. Kidneys were pale with interstitial nephritis [47]. Lung samples featured hemorrhage present in most lobes with mild to moderate multifocal interstitial pneumonitis, septal thickening, and multifocal edema [47]. These samples also had increased infiltration of lymphocytes and macrophages [47]. The adrenal cortex also featured mild to moderate inflammation and multifocal necrosis [47].

5.3. Rhesus Monkey (Rhesus Macaque) Model

Rhesus monkeys (*Rhesus macaques*) infected with the Josiah strain of LASV develop severe disease with prolonged viremia [44]. Succumbed animals developed disease signs by 7 dpi, including severe petechial rash, hiccups, lethargy, aphagia, huddled posture, constipation, conjunctivitis, anorexia, weight loss, decreased water intake/dehydration, facial and periorbital edema, bleeding from the gums and nares, cough, and a slight fever [44,48,49,54,55]. Fever persisted until death or a sudden hypothermia happened just before death approximately 10–14 dpi [44,49,54,55]. Subcutaneous inoculation with $10^{6.1}$ PFU of Josiah strain of LASV proved to be lethal in 60% of the animals [47]. Serologic analysis indicated antibody production by 10–12 dpi, although this was not correlated with viral clearance and animal recovery [44,49]. Elevated AST, ALT, and blood urea nitrogen (BUN) with a transient and moderate leukopenia was also noted [49,54,55]. Hematocrit, hemoglobin, fibronectin, and red blood cell counts decreased; platelet counts trended toward a decrease, although remained within the normal range [54,55]. Viremia appeared typically by 4–5 dpi with titers over 10^4 PFU/mL in lethally infected monkeys, significantly higher than those in survivors [49,54,55]. Viral loads were found in every organ tested including the adrenal glands, liver, lung, pancreas, brain, bone marrow, kidney, lymph nodes, spleen, muscle, heart, thymus, testis, salivary gland, urine, CSF, and intestines [44,49,55]. The highest titers were in the liver, spleen, and adrenal glands [55].

Gross pathological analysis indicated scattered petechial and visceral hemorrhage along with the presence of mild to moderate pleural effusions [44,48]. Liver and adrenal gland tissues presented with necrosis, with markers of regeneration of hepatocytes and a slight infiltration of inflammatory cells [44,48,49,55]. Interstitial pneumonia with edema, thickened alveolar septae, and pulmonary arteritis were present in the lung [44,48,49,55]. Spleen samples indicated lymphocytopenia and presence of viral antigens only in the red pulp [48,49]. Infected primates also developed mild to moderate interstitial and perivascular myocarditis and pericardial edema. Severe meningoencephalitis with significant perivascular cuffing was noted, albeit rarely [44,48]. Infiltration of erythrocytes and macrophages was noted in the small intestine. Lesions and a multifocal cortical interstitial mononuclear infiltrate were noted in the kidney [48,55]. Seventy-eight percent of infected primates developed lesions in the CNS with mild lymphocytic cuffing of the vessels of the brain, spinal cord, and meninges [48]. Twenty percent of primates suffered lymphocytic infiltration of the spiral ganglia; mild choriodoretinitis was also noted [48]. The arterial lesions, vasculitis, meningoencephalomyelitis and skeletal myositis observed in this monkey model were rarely, if at all, noted in human LF cases [44].

5.4. Cynomolgus Macaque Model

Josiah- or Z-132-infected "crab-eating" (cynomolgus) macaques developed a severe hemorrhagic disease with up to 100% of primates becoming moribund or dying between 11 and 18 dpi [38,39,50–53,56]. A study with the Soromba-R strain found two of three animals died (66% lethality) after infection and a prolonged time to euthanasia [39]. Infection with the Liberian LASV Z-132 strain was 100% lethal by 18 dpi [35]. Infection with 10^3 FFU AV strain featured only 67% lethality. All animals survived infection with 10^7 FFU of the AV strain, probably due to a high concentration of defective interfering (DI) viral particles in the higher dose [57]. Clinical signs, such as fever, weight loss, lethargy, dull appearance, reluctance to move/hypoactivity, anorexia, rashes, facial edema, hunched posture, ruffled fur, piloerection, bleeding from puncture sites, dehydration, epistaxis, acute respiratory syndrome, and mild to moderate depression appeared approximately 5-7 dpi, but might begin as early as 3 dpi [38,39,50–52,56–58]. Fever spiked between 7 and 10 dpi [39]. Viremia might start as early as 3–4 dpi, but was usually detectable 6–10 dpi, peaked 12–14 dpi, and continued to maintain high titers (up to 10^7 PFU/mL) until death or euthanasia [39,50,51,53,56,58]. Onset of fever was associated with detectable viremia. Survivors typically had a lower virus titer and cleared the virus by 28 dpi [50,57]. Survivors suffered neurological disorders such as tremors, reduced appetite, ataxia, convulsions/seizures, and unilateral or bilateral deafness [50,52,56,58]. Sixty-seven percent of the survivors developed hearing loss, which was thought to be driven by an immune-associated systemic vasculitis [50,56]. This hearing loss was present in all survivors of one study, presenting as unilateral or bilateral hearing loss [56].

Serologic analysis indicated elevated concentrations of AST, ALT, alkaline phosphatase (ALP), gamma-glutamyltransferase (GGT), total bilirubin (TBIL), and BUN as well as decreased concentrations of albumin, total protein, and amylase [38,39,50,51,58]. Transient lymphopenia, monocytopenia, neutropenia, and eosinopenia were also noticed at 4–10 dpi [38,39,50,51,58]. Platelet concentrations typically tended to decrease but remained within normal ranges, along with reduced hemoglobin, hematocrit, and creatinine concentrations [39,50,51,58]. The autoimmune markers C-reactive protein, antineutrophil cytoplasmic antibodies, and circulating immune complexes were also elevated in survivors with hearing loss [56]. Neutralizing antibodies were not detected in primates that succumbed to the infection but developed slowly in survivors approximately 14 dpi [50,56,57]. An early and strong T cell response was noticed in survivors [57]. Viral titers were detected at high levels in the spleen, lung, and liver, and at lower levels in the lymph nodes, kidney, and brain by 7 dpi [38,39,51,56–58].

Gross pathologic analysis revealed enlarged livers, spleens, adrenal glands, pancreas and lymph nodes, along with slight lung discoloration and pericardial effusion [38,39,57,58]. Lung samples featured mild to severe interstitial pneumonia with thickening of the alveolar septae [38,57,58]. Interestingly, although Soromba-R infections presented with a significantly less severe disease, the pathology of the lung was remarkable; 50–100% of lobes were reddened with lesions and extensive pulmonary infiltrations [38]. Liver samples were pale yellow and friable, featuring mild and multifocal portal hepatitis with random regions of necrosis [38,50,58]. Brain samples presented with meningoencephalitis in the frontal lobe, brainstem, and cerebellum with lesions. Neuritis was noted in the optic nerve [38,58]. Both lymph nodes and the white pulp of the spleen suffered follicular hyperplasia and mild lymphocytolysis. Spleens were also friable with fibrinous deposits in the red pulp [38,57,58]. Kidney samples appeared congested with mononuclear cell infiltrates [57,58]. Petechial hemorrhage and necrosis were noted on the bladder, while the ovaries and uterus were inflamed [57,58]. The thymus featured marked atrophy; myocarditis and necrotizing coronary arteritis were noted in the heart [58].

6. Surrogate Models of Lassa Fever

6.1. Pichindé Virus in Guinea Pigs

Pichindé virus (PICV) is a non-pathogenic, New World mammarenavirus isolated from cricetine rodents (*Oryzomys albigularis*) in Colombia, South America [59,60]. PICV infection of Strain 13 guinea pigs can cause Lassa-like disease and therefore has been used as a surrogate LASV model in BSL2 labs (Table 5) [61–63]. A minimum of four sequential passages of PICV in guinea pigs was required to result in 100% lethality [63,64]. Infected guinea pigs were hypoactive and lethargic, with ruffled fur, decreased food/water intake, rapid and shallow breathing, slobbering, and significant weight loss before becoming moribund [62,64]. Viremia appeared by 2 dpi and steadily increased until death at 16 dpi [62–64]. Infected guinea pigs featured extreme leukopenia beginning approximately 13 dpi and a transient neutrophilia [63]. Serologic findings included impaired platelet function, decreased activity of coagulation factors, and thrombocytopenia, decreased white blood cell concentrations and increased hematocrit [64]. AST concentrations were also elevated, starting from approximately 9 dpi [63]. Histologic analysis indicated pathological lesions in the liver, spleen, pancreas, lungs and gastrointestinal tract [61–64]. Scattered necrotic regions were found in lymphoid tissue and the bone marrow [64].

Table 5. Surrogate models of LASV infection.

Animal	Virus/Strain	Max. Dose	Route	Lethality	Signs of Disease	Affected Organs	Reference
Strain 13 (inbred) guinea pig	Pichindé virus	>3 PFU	SC	100%	hypoactivity, lethargy, ruffled fur, decreased appetite, rapid/shallow breathing, slobbering, weight loss, leukopenia, and transient neutrophilia	liver, spleen, pancreas, lung, gastrointestinal tract, lymphoid tissue, bone marrow	[61–64]
Hartley (outbred) guinea pig	Pichindé virus/P18	100 PFU	IP	100%	weight loss and fever	adrenal glands, lung, stomach, liver, brain, heart, spleen, pancreas, intestine, kidney, lymph node	[65,67]
	Pichindé virus/P2	10^4 PFU	IP	<100%	avirulent	none	[66]
	Pichindé virus/CoAn 4783	3000 PFU	IP	43%	weight loss and fever	cleared in survivors	[65]
LVG/Lak outbred golden hamsters	Pichindé virus	500 PFU	SC	0–100%	lethal infection up to 8 days post-birth; uncommon afterwards	spleen, liver, kidney	[68]
MHA/Lak inbred golden hamsters	Pichindé virus	3.5×10^6 PFU	IP	100%	lethal infection regardless of age	spleen, liver, kidney	[68]
Golden hamsters	Pirital virus	10^5 $TCID_{50}$	IP	>50%	hemorrhage, interstitial pneumonia, multifocal hepatic necrosis, splenic lymphoid depletion and necrosis	lung, liver, spleen	[69]
Rhesus monkeys	LCMV-WE	10^3 PFU	IV	100%	not listed	not listed	[70,71]
		10^8 PFU	IG [a]	20%	weight loss, elevated AST and ALT, thrombocytopenia, transient neutrophilia	liver	[72]

[a] IG: intragastic

Unlike Strain 13 guinea pigs, Hartley outbred guinea pigs did not uniformly succumb to infection by PICV CoAn 4763 strain [63,65]. The lethality was approximately 43% when animals were infected with 3000 PFU PICV CoAn 4763 [63]. Virus was cleared by 16 dpi in survivors [63]. When the CoAn 4763 strain passaged in Strain 13 guinea pigs for 18 passages, the resulting P18 strain was more virulent than the P2 strain, which was passaged only twice [65–67]. Infection with 100 PFU of the PICV P18 strain caused weight loss, fever and uniformly lethal infection in outbred guinea pigs [65–67]. Virus was present in almost all organs, with the highest titers in the adrenal glands, lungs, stomachs and livers [66]. Lower yet still notable titers were found in the brain [66]. P2-infected guinea pigs did not present with any detectable viral titer in any tested organs [66]. Additionally, P18 PICV-infected guinea pigs presented with a longer and more severe disease than their P2-infected counterparts [66]. The level of viremia was correlated with disease severity [66].

6.2. Pichindé Virus in Golden Hamsters

Pichindé virus infection also caused Lassa-like disease in Golden hamsters (*Mesocricetus auratus*) with various lethality depending on the virus strains (Table 5) [68]. The lethality could be 100% in new-born LVG/Lak outbred hamsters, and mortality was uncommon after 8 days post-birth. Peak viral titers in adults reached as high as 10^3 PFU/mL. MHA/Lak inbred hamsters demonstrated 100% lethality with as low as 35 PFU of virus regardless of ages [68]. Adults at 8 dpi developed viral titers over 10^8 PFU/mL. Both hamster models produced antibodies against the virus. Spleen, liver, and kidneys were the primary affected organs [68].

6.3. Pirital Virus in Golden Hamsters

Pirital virus, a non-human pathogenic New World mammarenavirus isolated from western Venezuela, causes a Lassa-like disease in Golden Hamsters [69]. These hamsters developed a severe disease and died approximately 7 dpi [69]. Interstitial pneumonia, multifocal hepatic necrosis, as well as splenic lymphoid depletion and necrosis were noted upon histologic analysis [69]. The brain, kidneys, and intestine were not significantly affected and there was no significant infiltration of inflammatory cells in the affected tissues [69]. Some of the infected hamsters presented with hemorrhagic signs from the mouth or puncture wounds. The clotting deficiency was noted in the collected blood samples, in which clotting rates were either non-existent or extremely slow [69].

6.4. Lymphocytic Choriomeningitis Virus (LCMV) in Rhesus Monkeys

The virulent WE strain of lymphocytic choriomeningitis virus (LCMV), a pathogenic Old World mammarenavirus, causes a uniformly lethal Lassa-like disease in rhesus monkeys infected intravenously (Table 5) [70]. Viremia was detected beginning at 4 dpi [70]. The liver especially was affected in this model, with significant gene expression changes noted [70,71]. However, of five primates infected intragastrically (IG), lethality only reached 20%, with only two of the monkeys becoming viremic [72]. Signs of disease included weight loss and serological analysis indicated elevated ALT and AST as well as thrombocytopenia, transient neutrophilia [72].

7. Summary

Animal models are essential for pathogenesis studies and LASV vaccine and antiviral developments. An ideal LF animal model should match the disease manifestation and progression, pathological changes, and the various pathogenicity of different strains in humans. Additionally, outbred animals with diverse genetic background have an advantage of mimicking infection in human populations. Other important factors include the immune-competency, the availability and the cost of the animals. The prototypic Josiah strain has been the most commonly used LASV strain in laboratory studies. However, the genetic diversity of LASV should also be considered when developing LF animal models.

The NHP models (Table 4), particularly "crab-eating" (cynomolgus) macaques, develop a disease very similar to clinical cases of LF and thus are excellent models for vaccine and antiviral evaluations as well as pathogenesis studies. However, the use of NHPs is extremely limited due to their relatively high cost, the difficulty of handling the animals, as well as the requirements for experienced staff and adequate space in high containment BSL4 facilities. Additionally, it is not easily feasible to perform NHP studies using large group sizes, making statistical significance difficult to ascertain.

Inbred Strain 13 guinea pigs are useful model animals, but the animals are not readily available and lack genetic diversity. Outbred Hartley guinea pigs are commercially available. However, the widely used Josiah strain must be adapted in guinea pigs in order to cause LF-like disease. PICV infection of Hartley guinea pigs can be used as a surrogate animal model of LF. Using the clinical LASV

LF2384 isolate, which was isolated from a fatal case and has experienced minimal passaging in the laboratory, uniformly lethality can be achieved in Hartley guinea pigs without species-specific adaptation. Although further characterization is required, this new model shows much potential as a relevant and relatively inexpensive rodent model that combines the advantages of diverse genetic background, immunocompetency as well as the convenience of the animal's small size and large numbers that can be used in an experiment, which can ensure the rigor and reproducibility of the studies. However, one limitation of using guinea pigs is the lack of available laboratory reagents and a collection of genetically modified animals for immunological and related studies. Nevertheless, guinea pig models could be ideal for vaccine and antiviral screening and potentially pathogenesis studies. A summary of guinea pig LF disease manifestations and pathologies can be found in Table 3.

Immune-competent laboratory mice are generally resistant to LASV infection (Table 2). The STAT1$^{-/-}$ mouse model is the only known animal model for studying LASV-associated hearing loss. This new mouse model has been used in studies on the pathogenesis and immunology of LF, which indicate an immunopathological mechanism of LF. This mouse model may be useful in initial vaccine and antiviral drug screening, as it is a lethal model of infection. However, its immune-incompetency should be considered, as deficiency in interferon signaling may have negative effects on such studies [73,74].

With the increased fatality of LF in the most recent 2018–2019 outbreaks, there is an urgent need for the rapid development of vaccines and antivirals. Development of small animal models that resemble human disease is crucial to facilitate vaccine and therapeutic testing. The best option at the current stage seems to be performing initial screening in lethal rodent models, such as the aforementioned STAT1$^{-/-}$ mouse model and the newly developed LF2384/outbred Hartley guinea pig model, followed by validation of promising candidates in NHPs. Additionally, the STAT1$^{-/-}$ model is useful as a new platform for investigating the mechanism of LF-associated hearing loss, which affects approximately one third of survivors.

Author Contributions: Review conceptualization and organization were conducted by all authors. The original manuscript was prepared by R.A.S. Manuscript editing was performed by all authors. All authors have read and agree to the published version of the manuscript.

Funding: R.A.S. was supported by the Institute for Translational Sciences at the University of Texas Medical Branch, which is supported in part and by the Clinical and Translational Science Award NRSA (TL1) Training Core (TL1TR001440) from the National Center for Advancing Translational Sciences at the National Institutes of Health. Work in the Paessler laboratory was supported in parts by Public Health Service grants RO1AI093445 and RO1AI129198 and the John. S. Dunn Distinguished Chair in Biodefense endowment. Work in the Ly lab was supported in parts by the Public Health Service grant R01AI131586 and by funds from the USDA National Institute of Food and Agriculture (USDA-NIFA) and from the Minnesota Agricultural Experiment Station. C.H. was supported by UTMB Commitment Fund P84373.

Acknowledgments: We apologize for any works that we were unable to include due to the constraints of the review. The authors would like to thank Junki Maruyama for consultation over the course of writing. C.H. would like to acknowledge the Galveston National Laboratory (supported by the Public Health Service award 5UC7AI094660) for support of his research activity.

Conflicts of Interest: The authors declare no conflict of interest.

References

1. Günther, S.; Lenz, O. Lassa fever. *Br. Med. J.* **1972**, *4*, 253–254. Available online: https://www.ncbi.nlm.nih.gov/pmc/articles/PMC1788780/ (accessed on 14 June 2019).
2. Centers for Disease Control and Prevention. Lassa Fever. 2019. Available online: https://www.cdc.gov/vhf/lassa/index.html (accessed on 15 June 2019).
3. Frame, J.D.; Baldwin, J.M., Jr.; Gocke, D.J.; Troup, J.M. Lassa fever, a new virus disease of man from West Africa. I. Clinical description and pathological findings. *Am. J. Trop. Med. Hyg.* **1970**, *19*, 670–676. [CrossRef] [PubMed]
4. Olayemi, A.; Oyeyiola, A.; Obadare, A.; Igbokwe, J.; Adesina, A.S.; Onwe, F.; Ukwaja, K.N.; Ajayi, N.A.; Rieger, T.; Gunther, S.; et al. Widespread arenavirus occurrence and seroprevalence in small mammals, Nigeria. *Parasit Vectors* **2018**, *11*, 416. [CrossRef]

5. Andersen, K.G.; Shapiro, B.J.; Matranga, C.B.; Sealfon, R.; Lin, A.E.; Moses, L.M.; Folarin, O.A.; Goba, A.; Odia, I.; Ehiane, P.E.; et al. Clinical Sequencing Uncovers Origins and Evolution of Lassa Virus. *Cell* **2015**, *162*, 738–750. [CrossRef]
6. Manning, J.T.; Forrester, N.; Paessler, S. Lassa virus isolates from Mali and the Ivory Coast represent an emerging fifth lineage. *Front. Microbiol.* **2015**, *6*, 1037. [CrossRef]
7. Ehichioya, D.U.; Dellicour, S.; Pahlmann, M.; Rieger, T.; Oestereich, L.; Becker-Ziaja, B.; Cadar, D.; Ighodalo, Y.; Olokor, T.; Omomoh, E.; et al. Phylogeography of Lassa Virus in Nigeria. *J. Virol.* **2019**, *93*. [CrossRef]
8. Yun, N.E.; Ronca, S.; Tamura, A.; Koma, T.; Seregin, A.V.; Dineley, K.T.; Miller, M.; Cook, R.; Shimizu, N.; Walker, A.G.; et al. Animal Model of Sensorineural Hearing Loss Associated with Lassa Virus Infection. *J. Virol.* **2015**, *90*, 2920–2927. [CrossRef]
9. Welch, S.R.; Scholte, F.E.M.; Albariño, C.G.; Kainulainen, M.H.; Coleman-McCray, J.D.; Guerrero, L.W.; Chakrabarti, A.K.; Klena, J.D.; Nichol, S.T.; Spengler, J.R.; et al. The S Genome Segment Is Sufficient to Maintain Pathogenicity in Intra-Clade Lassa Virus Reassortants in a Guinea Pig Model. *Front. Cell. Infect. Microbiol.* **2018**, *8*, 240. [CrossRef]
10. Ibekwe, T.S.; Okokhere, P.O.; Asogun, D.; Blackie, F.F.; Nwegbu, M.M.; Wahab, K.W.; Omilabu, S.A.; Akpede, G.O. Early-onset sensorineural hearing loss in Lassa fever. *Eur. Arch. Otorhinolaryngol.* **2011**, *268*, 197–201. [CrossRef]
11. Dan-Nwafor, C.C.; Furuse, Y.; Ilori, E.A.; Ipadeola, O.; Akabike, K.O.; Ahumibe, A.; Ukponu, W.; Bakare, L.; Okwor, T.J.; Joseph, G.; et al. Measures to control protracted large Lassa fever outbreak in Nigeria, 1 January to 28 April 2019. *Euro. Surveill.* **2019**, *24*. [CrossRef]
12. World Health Organization. On the Frontlines of the Fight against Lassa Fever in Nigeria. 2018. Available online: http://www.who.int/features/2018/lassa-fever-nigeria/en/ (accessed on 15 June 2019).
13. Nigeria Centers for Disease Control. 2018 Lassa Fever Outbreak in Nigeria. 2018. Available online: https://ncdc.gov.ng/themes/common/files/sitreps/00235292b8a3f55c01f9ea2eb15c8d3a.pdf (accessed on 15 June 2019).
14. World Health Organization. Emergencies Preparedness, Response Lassa Fever. 2019. Available online: https://www.who.int/csr/don/archive/disease/lassa_fever/en/ (accessed on 16 June 2019).
15. McCormick, J.B.; King, I.J.; Webb, P.A.; Scribner, C.L.; Craven, R.B.; Johnson, K.M.; Elliott, L.H.; Belmont-Williams, R. Lassa fever. Effective therapy with ribavirin. *N. Engl. J. Med.* **1986**, *314*, 20–26. [CrossRef]
16. Mustapha, A. Lassa fever: Unveiling the misery of the Nigerian health worker. *Ann. Nigerian. Med.* **2017**, *11*, 1–5.
17. Walker, D.H.; McCormick, J.B.; Johnson, K.M.; Webb, P.A.; Komba-Kono, G.; Elliott, L.H.; Gardner, J.J. Pathologic and virologic study of fatal Lassa fever in man. *Am. J. Pathol.* **1982**, *107*, 349–356.
18. Mateer, E.J.; Huang, C.; Shehu, N.Y.; Paessler, S. Lassa fever-induced sensorineural hearing loss: A neglected public health and social burden. *PLoS Negl. Trop. Dis.* **2018**, *12*, e0006187. [CrossRef]
19. Cummins, D.; McCormick, J.B.; Bennett, D.; Samba, J.A.; Farrar, B.; Machin, S.J.; Fisher-Hoch, S.P. Acute sensorineural deafness in Lassa fever. *JAMA* **1990**, *264*, 2093–2096. [CrossRef]
20. Price, M.E.; Fisher-Hoch, S.P.; Craven, R.B.; McCormick, J.B. A prospective study of maternal and fetal outcome in acute Lassa fever infection during pregnancy. *BMJ* **1988**, *297*, 584–587. [CrossRef]
21. Dunmade, A.D.; Segun-Busari, S.; Olajide, T.G.; Ologe, F.E. Profound bilateral sensorineural hearing loss in nigerian children: Any shift in etiology? *J. Deaf Stud. Deaf Educ.* **2007**, *12*, 112–118. [CrossRef]
22. Khan, S.H.; Goba, A.; Chu, M.; Roth, C.; Healing, T.; Marx, A.; Fair, J.; Guttieri, M.C.; Ferro, P.; Imes, T.; et al. New opportunities for field research on the pathogenesis and treatment of Lassa fever. *Antiviral. Res.* **2008**, *78*, 103–115. [CrossRef]
23. Johnson, K.M.; McCormick, J.B.; Webb, P.A.; Smith, E.S.; Elliott, L.H.; King, I.J. Clinical virology of Lassa fever in hospitalized patients. *J. Infect. Dis.* **1987**, *155*, 456–464. [CrossRef]
24. Winn, W.C., Jr.; Walker, D.H. The pathology of human Lassa fever. *Bull. World Health Organ.* **1975**, *52*, 535–545.
25. Walker, D.H.; Wulff, H.; Lange, J.V.; Murphy, F.A. Comparative pathology of Lassa virus infection in monkeys, guinea-pigs, and *Mastomys natalensis*. *Bull. World Health Organ.* **1975**, *52*, 523–534. [PubMed]
26. Granjon, L.; Duplantier, J.-M.; Catalan, J.; Britton-Davidian, J. Systematics of the genus Mastomys (Thomas, 1915) (Rodentia: Muridae): A review. *Belg. J. Zool.* **1997**, *127*, 7–18.
27. Rieger, T.; Merkler, D.; Gunther, S. Infection of type I interferon receptor-deficient mice with various old world arenaviruses: A model for studying virulence and host species barriers. *PLoS One* **2013**, *8*, e72290. [CrossRef]

28. Yun, N.E.; Seregin, A.V.; Walker, D.H.; Popov, V.L.; Walker, A.G.; Smith, J.N.; Miller, M.; de la Torre, J.C.; Smith, J.K.; Borisevich, V.; et al. Mice lacking functional STAT1 are highly susceptible to lethal infection with Lassa virus. *J. Virol.* **2013**, *87*, 10908–10911. [CrossRef]
29. Oestereich, L.; Lüdtke, A.; Ruibal, P.; Pallasch, E.; Kerber, R.; Rieger, T.; Wurr, S.; Bockholt, S.; Pérez-Girón, J.V.; Krasemann, S.; et al. Chimeric Mice with Competent Hematopoietic Immunity Reproduce Key Features of Severe Lassa Fever. *PLoS Pathog.* **2016**, *12*, e1005656. [CrossRef]
30. Yun, N.E.; Poussard, A.L.; Seregin, A.V.; Walker, A.G.; Smith, J.K.; Aronson, J.F.; Smith, J.N.; Soong, L.; Paessler, S. Functional interferon system is required for clearance of lassa virus. *J. Virol.* **2012**, *86*, 3389–3392. [CrossRef]
31. Oestereich, L.; Rieger, T.; Ludtke, A.; Ruibal, P.; Wurr, S.; Pallasch, E.; Bockholt, S.; Krasemann, S.; Muñoz-Fontela, C.; Gunther, S. Efficacy of Favipiravir Alone and in Combination With Ribavirin in a Lethal, Immunocompetent Mouse Model of Lassa Fever. *J. Infect. Dis.* **2016**, *213*, 934–938. [CrossRef]
32. Uckun, F.M.; Petkevich, A.S.; Vassilev, A.O.; Tibbles, H.E.; Titov, L. Stampidine prevents mortality in an experimental mouse model of viral hemorrhagic fever caused by lassa virus. *BMC Infect. Dis.* **2004**, *4*, 1. [CrossRef]
33. Flatz, L.; Rieger, T.; Merkler, D.; Bergthaler, A.; Regen, T.; Schedensack, M.; Bestmann, L.; Verschoor, A.; Kreutzfeldt, M.; Bruck, W.; et al. T cell-dependence of Lassa fever pathogenesis. *PLoS Pathog.* **2010**, *6*, e1000836. [CrossRef]
34. Jahrling, P.B.; Smith, S.; Hesse, R.A.; Rhoderick, J.B. Pathogenesis of Lassa virus infection in guinea pigs. *Infect. Immun.* **1982**, *37*, 771–778. [CrossRef]
35. Bell, T.M.; Shaia, C.I.; Bearss, J.J.; Mattix, M.E.; Koistinen, K.A.; Honnold, S.P.; Zeng, X.; Blancett, C.D.; Donnelly, G.C.; Shamblin, J.D.; et al. Temporal Progression of Lesions in Guinea Pigs Infected With Lassa Virus. *Vet. Pathol.* **2017**, *54*, 549–562. [CrossRef] [PubMed]
36. Gary, J.M.; Welch, S.R.; Ritter, J.M.; Coleman-McCray, J.; Huynh, T.; Kainulainen, M.H.; Bollweg, B.C.; Parihar, V.; Nichol, S.T.; Zaki, S.R.; et al. Lassa Virus Targeting of Anterior Uvea and Endothelium of Cornea and Conjunctiva in Eye of Guinea Pig Model. *Emerg. Infect. Dis.* **2019**, *25*, 865–874. [CrossRef] [PubMed]
37. Cashman, K.A.; Smith, M.A.; Twenhafel, N.A.; Larson, R.A.; Jones, K.F.; Allen, R.D., 3rd; Dai, D.; Chinsangaram, J.; Bolken, T.C.; Hruby, D.E.; et al. Evaluation of Lassa antiviral compound ST-193 in a guinea pig model. *Antiviral. Res.* **2011**, *90*, 70–79. [CrossRef] [PubMed]
38. Safronetz, D.; Mire, C.; Rosenke, K.; Feldmann, F.; Haddock, E.; Geisbert, T.; Feldmann, H. A recombinant vesicular stomatitis virus-based Lassa fever vaccine protects guinea pigs and macaques against challenge with geographically and genetically distinct Lassa viruses. *PLoS Negl. Trop. Dis.* **2015**, *9*, e0003736. [CrossRef] [PubMed]
39. Safronetz, D.; Strong, J.E.; Feldmann, F.; Haddock, E.; Sogoba, N.; Brining, D.; Geisbert, T.W.; Scott, D.P.; Feldmann, H. A recently isolated Lassa virus from Mali demonstrates atypical clinical disease manifestations and decreased virulence in cynomolgus macaques. *J. Infect. Dis.* **2013**, *207*, 1316–1327. [CrossRef] [PubMed]
40. Cross, R.W.; Mire, C.E.; Branco, L.M.; Geisbert, J.B.; Rowland, M.M.; Heinrich, M.L.; Goba, A.; Momoh, M.; Grant, D.S.; Fullah, M.; et al. Treatment of Lassa virus infection in outbred guinea pigs with first-in-class human monoclonal antibodies. *Antiviral. Res.* **2016**, *133*, 218–222. [CrossRef]
41. Safronetz, D.; Rosenke, K.; Westover, J.B.; Martellaro, C.; Okumura, A.; Furuta, Y.; Geisbert, J.; Saturday, G.; Komeno, T.; Geisbert, T.W.; et al. The broad-spectrum antiviral favipiravir protects guinea pigs from lethal Lassa virus infection post-disease onset. *Sci. Rep.* **2015**, *5*, 14775. [CrossRef]
42. Stein, D.R.; Warner, B.M.; Soule, G.; Tierney, K.; Frost, K.L.; Booth, S.; Safronetz, D. A recombinant vesicular stomatitis-based Lassa fever vaccine elicits rapid and long-term protection from lethal Lassa virus infection in guinea pigs. *NPJ Vaccines* **2019**, *4*, 8. [CrossRef]
43. Maruyama, J.; Mateer, E.J.; Manning, J.T.; Sattler, R.; Seregin, A.V.; Bukreyeva, N.; Jones, F.R.; Balint, J.P.; Gabitzsch, E.S.; Huang, C.; et al. Adenoviral vector-based vaccine is fully protective against lethal Lassa fever challenge in Hartley guinea pigs. *Vaccine* **2019**, *37*, 6824–6831. [CrossRef]
44. Walker, D.H.; Johnson, K.M.; Lange, J.V.; Gardner, J.J.; Kiley, M.P.; McCormick, J.B. Experimental infection of rhesus monkeys with Lassa virus and a closely related arenavirus, Mozambique virus. *J. Infect. Dis.* **1982**, *146*, 360–368. [CrossRef] [PubMed]
45. Maruyama, J.; Manning, J.T.; Mateer, E.J.; Sattler, R.; Bukreyeva, N.; Huang, C.; Paessler, S. Lethal Infection of Lassa Virus Isolated from a Human Clinical Sample in Outbred Guinea Pigs without Adaptation. *mSphere* **2019**, *4*. [CrossRef] [PubMed]
46. Walker, D.H.; Wulff, H.; Murphy, F.A. Experimental Lassa virus infection in the squirrel monkey. *Am. J. Pathol.* **1975**, *80*, 261–278. [PubMed]

47. Carrion, R., Jr.; Brasky, K.; Mansfield, K.; Johnson, C.; Gonzales, M.; Ticer, A.; Lukashevich, I.; Tardif, S.; Patterson, J. Lassa virus infection in experimentally infected marmosets: Liver pathology and immunophenotypic alterations in target tissues. *J. Virol.* **2007**, *81*, 6482–6490. [CrossRef] [PubMed]
48. Callis, R.T.; Jahrling, P.B.; DePaoli, A. Pathology of Lassa virus infection in the rhesus monkey. *Am. J. Trop. Med. Hyg.* **1982**, *31*, 1038–1045. [CrossRef] [PubMed]
49. Jahrling, P.B.; Hesse, R.A.; Eddy, G.A.; Johnson, K.M.; Callis, R.T.; Stephen, E.L. Lassa virus infection of rhesus monkeys: Pathogenesis and treatment with ribavirin. *J. Infect. Dis.* **1980**, *141*, 580–589. [CrossRef]
50. Cashman, K.A.; Wilkinson, E.R.; Shaia, C.I.; Facemire, P.R.; Bell, T.M.; Bearss, J.J.; Shamblin, J.D.; Wollen, S.E.; Broderick, K.E.; Sardesai, N.Y.; et al. A DNA vaccine delivered by dermal electroporation fully protects cynomolgus macaques against Lassa fever. *Hum. Vaccin. Immunother.* **2017**, *13*, 2902–2911. [CrossRef]
51. Geisbert, T.W.; Jones, S.; Fritz, E.A.; Shurtleff, A.C.; Geisbert, J.B.; Liebscher, R.; Grolla, A.; Ströher, U.; Fernando, L.; Daddario, K.M.; et al. Development of a new vaccine for the prevention of Lassa fever. *PLoS Med.* **2005**, *2*, e183. [CrossRef]
52. Jiang, J.; Banglore, P.; Cashman, K.A.; Schmaljohn, C.S.; Schultheis, K.; Pugh, H.; Nguyen, J.; Humeau, L.M.; Broderick, K.E.; Ramos, S.J. Immunogenicity of a protective intradermal DNA vaccine against lassa virus in cynomolgus macaques. *Hum. Vaccin. Immunother.* **2019**, *15*, 2066–2074. [CrossRef]
53. Mire, C.E.; Cross, R.W.; Geisbert, J.B.; Borisevich, V.; Agans, K.N.; Deer, D.J.; Heinrich, M.L.; Rowland, M.M.; Goba, A.; Momoh, M.; et al. Human-monoclonal-antibody therapy protects nonhuman primates against advanced Lassa fever. *Nat. Med.* **2017**, *23*, 1146–1149. [CrossRef]
54. Fisher-Hoch, S.P.; Mitchell, S.W.; Sasso, D.R.; Lange, J.V.; Ramsey, R.; McCormick, J.B. Physiological and immunologic disturbances associated with shock in a primate model of Lassa fever. *J. Infect. Dis.* **1987**, *155*, 465–474. [CrossRef]
55. Lange, J.V.; Mitchell, S.W.; McCormick, J.B.; Walker, D.H.; Evatt, B.L.; Ramsey, R.R. Kinetic study of platelets and fibrinogen in Lassa virus-infected monkeys and early pathologic events in Mopeia virus-infected monkeys. *Am. J. Trop. Med. Hyg.* **1985**, *34*, 999–1007. [CrossRef] [PubMed]
56. Cashman, K.A.; Wilkinson, E.R.; Zeng, X.; Cardile, A.P.; Facemire, P.R.; Bell, T.M.; Bearss, J.J.; Shaia, C.I.; Schmaljohn, C.S. Immune-Mediated Systemic Vasculitis as the Proposed Cause of Sudden-Onset Sensorineural Hearing Loss following Lassa Virus Exposure in Cynomolgus Macaques. *mBio* **2018**, *9*. [CrossRef] [PubMed]
57. Baize, S.; Marianneau, P.; Loth, P.; Reynard, S.; Journeaux, A.; Chevallier, M.; Tordo, N.; Deubel, V.; Contamin, H. Early and strong immune responses are associated with control of viral replication and recovery in lassa virus-infected cynomolgus monkeys. *J. Virol.* **2009**, *83*, 5890–5903. [CrossRef] [PubMed]
58. Hensley, L.E.; Smith, M.A.; Geisbert, J.B.; Fritz, E.A.; Daddario-DiCaprio, K.M.; Larsen, T.; Geisbert, T.W. Pathogenesis of Lassa fever in cynomolgus macaques. *Virol. J.* **2011**, *8*, 205. [CrossRef]
59. Buchmeier, M.; Adam, E.; Rawls, W.E. Serological evidence of infection by Pichindé virus among laboratory workers. *Infect. Immun.* **1974**, *9*, 821–823. [CrossRef]
60. Trapido, H.; Sanmartin, C. Pichindé virus, a new virus of the Tacaribe group from Colombia. *Am. J. Trop. Med. Hyg.* **1971**, *20*, 631–641. [CrossRef]
61. Aronson, J.F.; Herzog, N.K.; Jerrells, T.R. Pathological and virological features of arenavirus disease in guinea pigs. Comparison of two Pichindé virus strains. *Am. J. Pathol.* **1994**, *145*, 228–235.
62. Connolly, B.M.; Jenson, A.B.; Peters, C.J.; Geyer, S.J.; Barth, J.F.; McPherson, R.A. Pathogenesis of Pichindé virus infection in strain 13 guinea pigs: An immunocytochemical, virologic, and clinical chemistry study. *Am. J. Trop. Med. Hyg.* **1993**, *49*, 10–24. [CrossRef]
63. Jahrling, P.B.; Hesse, R.A.; Rhoderick, J.B.; Elwell, M.A.; Moe, J.B. Pathogenesis of a pichindé virus strain adapted to produce lethal infections in guinea pigs. *Infect. Immun.* **1981**, *32*, 872–880. [CrossRef]
64. Cosgriff, T.M.; Jahrling, P.B.; Chen, J.P.; Hodgson, L.A.; Lewis, R.M.; Green, D.E.; Smith, J.I. Studies of the coagulation system in arenaviral hemorrhagic fever: Experimental infection of strain 13 guinea pigs with Pichindé virus. *Am. J. Trop. Med. Hyg.* **1987**, *36*, 416–423. [CrossRef]
65. Zhang, L.; Marriott, K.; Aronson, J.F. Sequence analysis of the small RNA segment of guinea pig-passaged Pichindé virus variants. *Am. J. Trop. Med. Hyg.* **1999**, *61*, 220–225. [CrossRef] [PubMed]
66. Lan, S.; McLay Schelde, L.; Wang, J.; Kumar, N.; Ly, H.; Liang, Y. Development of infectious clones for virulent and avirulent pichindé viruses: A model virus to study arenavirus-induced hemorrhagic fevers. *J. Virol.* **2009**, *83*, 6357–6362. [CrossRef] [PubMed]

67. Zhang, L.; Marriott, K.A.; Harnish, D.G.; Aronson, J.F. Reassortant analysis of guinea pig virulence of pichindé virus variants. *Virology* **2001**, *290*, 30–38. [CrossRef]
68. Buchmeier, M.J.; Rawls, W.E. Variation between strains of hamsters in the lethality of Pichindé virus infections. *Infect. Immun.* **1977**, *16*, 413–421. [CrossRef] [PubMed]
69. Xiao, S.Y.; Zhang, H.; Yang, Y.; Tesh, R.B. Pirital virus (*Arenaviridae*) infection in the syrian golden hamster, Mesocricetus auratus: A new animal model for arenaviral hemorrhagic fever. *Am. J. Trop. Med. Hyg.* **2001**, *64*, 111–118. [CrossRef] [PubMed]
70. Djavani, M.M.; Crasta, O.R.; Zapata, J.C.; Fei, Z.; Folkerts, O.; Sobral, B.; Swindells, M.; Bryant, J.; Davis, H.; Pauza, C.D.; et al. Early blood profiles of virus infection in a monkey model for Lassa fever. *J. Virol.* **2007**, *81*, 7960–7973. [CrossRef] [PubMed]
71. Djavani, M.; Crasta, O.R.; Zhang, Y.; Zapata, J.C.; Sobral, B.; Lechner, M.G.; Bryant, J.; Davis, H.; Salvato, M.S. Gene expression in primate liver during viral hemorrhagic fever. *Virol. J.* **2009**, *6*, 20. [CrossRef]
72. Rodas, J.D.; Lukashevich, I.S.; Zapata, J.C.; Cairo, C.; Tikhonov, I.; Djavani, M.; Pauza, C.D.; Salvato, M.S. Mucosal arenavirus infection of primates can protect them from lethal hemorrhagic fever. *J. Med. Virol.* **2004**, *72*, 424–435. [CrossRef]
73. Clarke, E.C.; Bradfute, S.B. The use of mice lacking type I or both type I and type II interferon responses in research on hemorrhagic fever viruses. Part 1: Potential effects on adaptive immunity and response to vaccination. *Antiviral. Res.* **2020**, *174*, 104703. [CrossRef] [PubMed]
74. Zivcec, M.; Spiropoulou, C.F.; Spengler, J.R. The use of mice lacking type I or both type I and type II interferon responses in research on hemorrhagic fever viruses. Part 2: Vaccine efficacy studies. *Antiviral. Res.* **2020**, *174*, 104702. [CrossRef]

pathogens

MDPI

Review

Virus–Host Interactions Involved in Lassa Virus Entry and Genome Replication

María Eugenia Loureiro *, Alejandra D'Antuono and Nora López

Centro de Virología Animal (CEVAN), CONICET-SENASA, Av Sir Alexander Fleming 1653, Martínez, Provincia de Buenos Aires B1640CSI, Argentina; adantuono@gmail.com (A.D.); noramlopar@gmail.com (N.L.)
* Correspondence: eugenialoureiro@yahoo.com.ar; Tel.: +54-11-4105-4100

Received: 21 December 2018; Accepted: 26 January 2019; Published: 29 January 2019

Abstract: Lassa virus (LASV) is the causative agent of Lassa fever, a human hemorrhagic disease associated with high mortality and morbidity rates, particularly prevalent in West Africa. Over the past few years, a significant amount of novel information has been provided on cellular factors that are determinant elements playing a role in arenavirus multiplication. In this review, we focus on host proteins that intersect with the initial steps of the LASV replication cycle: virus entry and genome replication. A better understanding of relevant virus–host interactions essential for sustaining these critical steps may help to identify possible targets for the rational design of novel therapeutic approaches against LASV and other arenaviruses that cause severe human disease.

Keywords: Lassa fever; arenavirus; LASV; virus–host interactions; entry; replication

1. Introduction

The *Arenaviridae* family includes viruses carried by mammalian hosts, classified in the Mammarenavirus genus, and members that infect reptilian hosts, which belong to the Reptarenavirus and Hartmanivirus genera [1]. Mammarenaviruses comprise 35 currently recognized species that are classified into two main groups, Old World (OW) and New World (NW) viruses. Within the NW group, viruses are divided into Clade A, Clade A-recombinant (Clade D), Clade B, and Clade C, according to their phylogenetic relationships. Clade B includes the apathogenic Tacaribe virus (TCRV), along with the known South American pathogens that produce severe hemorrhagic disease in humans: Junín virus (JUNV), the causative agent of Argentine hemorrhagic fever; and Machupo, Chapare, Guanarito, and Sabia viruses. OW mammarenaviruses include the prototypic lymphocytic choriomeningitis virus (LCMV), of worldwide distribution, and other viruses endemic to the African continent such as Mopeia (MOPV), Lujo (LUJV), and Lassa virus (LASV). LASV is the causative agent of Lassa fever (LF), a human hemorrhagic disease transmitted through contact with infected rodents (*Mastomys* spp.) that is particularly prevalent in Nigeria, Liberia, Sierra Leone, and Guinea. After infection, an average incubation time of 10 days is usually followed by general flu-like symptoms, including fever, malaise, and headache. Hemorrhagic and/or neurologic involvement can be associated with severe cases of LF [2]. Up to 500,000 infections and >5000 deaths occur every year, with mortality rates which can rise up to 50% in hospitalized patients, 90% in women in the last month of pregnancy, and nearly 100% mortality in fetuses [3]. Neurological sequelae including deafness are common features in LF survivors [4,5].

Arenaviruses are enveloped viruses with a negative-sense RNA genome, consisting of two single-stranded segments named S (ca. 3.4 kb) and L (ca. 7.2 kb), each encoding two proteins with an ambisense strategy for expression. The S segment encodes the nucleoprotein (NP) and the precursor of the envelope glycoprotein complex (GPC), while the L segment encodes the viral RNA-dependent RNA polymerase (L) and a matrix protein (Z) that is involved in virus assembly and budding [6].

The open reading frames, in opposite orientations, are separated by a noncoding intergenic region predicted to fold into strong stem-loop structures [7].

GPC is expressed as a single precursor polypeptide that is cleaved twice by cellular proteases to generate a stable signal peptide (SSP), a receptor-binding subunit (GP1), and a trans-membrane fusion subunit (GP2). Both the peripheral GP1 and the SSP remain noncovalently associated with GP2, and assemble into the trimeric glycoprotein (GP) complex that mediates receptor recognition and fusion of the viral and host cell membranes [8–10].

NP is the most abundant viral protein both in virions and infected cells, and plays critical roles during arenavirus life cycle. NP associates tightly with the viral genomic and antigenomic RNAs forming ribonucleoprotein (RNP) complexes called nucleocapsids. Nucleocapsids bind the L polymerase, constituting the biologically active units for transcription of subgenomic viral mRNAs and for viral genome replication [11–13]. In addition, NP interacts with the Z matrix protein and contributes to the packaging of RNPs into viral particles during virion morphogenesis [14–16]. Crystallographic studies revealed that LASV NP is organized in two distinct domains [17]. The N-terminal domain contains a basic crevice, initially proposed to be an m7GTP cap binding site and later reported to function in binding RNA [17,18]. The C-terminal domain of NP harbors a functional 3′-5′ exoribonuclease activity of the DExD/H-box protein family that has been shown to oppose the host type I interferon (IFN-I)-mediated immune response during viral infection. In this regard, NP is capable of degrading small viral doubled-stranded RNA fragments that could function as pathogen-associated molecular patterns, to prevent their recognition by cellular pattern recognition receptors (PRRs) [17,19–21]. In addition, the role of NP in the negative regulation of IFN-I production has been linked to its ability to prevent the nuclear translocation and transcriptional activity of the nuclear factor kappa B (NF-kB), and its direct association with the retinoic acid-inducible gene I (RIG-I) and I-kappa-B kinase epsilon (IKKε), thereby inhibiting the activation and nuclear translocation of the interferon regulatory factor 3 (IRF-3) [22–24].

Following arenavirus entry, nucleocapsids are delivered into the cytoplasm of the host cell where transcription and replication of viral RNA segments occur. The arenavirus Z protein directs the assembly and budding of infectious particles from the plasma membrane, co-opting proteins from the endosomal sorting complexes required for transport (ESCRT) that facilitate virus egress [25].

Over the past few years, a significant amount of novel information has accrued regarding cellular proteins that play a role in the arenavirus life cycle, including in pathogenesis, immune evasion and virus entry and egress [25–28]. Here, we summarize current knowledge on host factors that are involved in LASV entry and discuss factors crucial for LASV RNA replication. Deepening the knowledge about relevant virus-host interactions essential for sustaining these early critical steps may help identify possible targets for the rational design of novel therapeutic approaches against LASV and other arenaviruses that cause severe human disease.

2. Virus–Host Interactions Involved in LASV Entry

2.1. α-Dystroglycan (α-DG) Is the Principal Receptor for LASV Entry

Arenaviruses primarily attach to cells by binding of their surface GP to specific receptor/entry factors at the plasma membrane of host cells. α-DG was the first entry receptor discovered for LASV, as well as for other OW and for Clade C NW arenaviruses [29,30], and its interaction with GP has been widely characterized [31]. DG is expressed as a precursor and proteolytically cleaved to generate the mature α and β subunits that together serve as a molecular bridge between the extracellular matrix and the cytoplasm [32–35]. α-DG is found in the extracellular compartment, where it binds components such as laminin, and requires *O*-glycosylation to perform its biological functions [36,37], whereas the transmembrane β subunit (β-DG) docks to the cytoskeleton by associating to the cytoplasmic adaptor proteins dystrophin and utrophin [35,38,39]. DG is expressed in most cell types, but its expression patterns and glycosylation levels differ depending on the tissue [34,35].

Further reports on arenavirus biology provide evidence that the α-DG receptor requires a specific type of glycosylation for efficient virus attachment; in particular, *O*-mannosylation, rarely found in mammals [40,41]. LASV tightly binds to the "matriglycan" platform displayed on α-DG, a polymer composed of 3-xylose-α1, 3-glucuronic acid-β1 (Xylα1-3GlcAβ1-3) disaccharide repeats, which is linked to α-DG through phosphorylated *O*-mannose. Like-acetylglucosaminyltransferase (LARGE) is required for the attachment of ligand-binding moieties to phosphorylated *O*-mannose on α-DG [42]. Moreover, the recent determination of the crystal structure of the mature LASV and LCMV GPs in prefusion conformation demonstrates that the GP ectodomain engages matriglycan via multiple contacts, with a close similarity to the molecular mechanisms driving α-DG recognition of host extracellular matrix (ECM) proteins [43,44]. Therefore, it is reasonable to conceive that LASV would mimic the behavior of different host ECMs that normally interact with glycosylated membrane receptors to gain access to the cell. Indeed, post-translational modification of α-DG by the glycosyltransferase LARGE is required for both efficient LASV infection and laminin binding [45–47]. Mutagenesis and functional studies further identified two threonine (Thr) residues (Thr317 and Thr319) within a highly conserved amino acid motif in α-DG that play a key role in LARGE-mediated α-DG modification, and are required for recognition by LASV GP and laminin [48]. These findings further support the idea that arenaviruses displaying high affinity for α-DG may be able to compete with host ligands and displace them from the receptor to infiltrate the cell [45,48]. Thereafter, upon receptor recognition, the encounter of cellular α-DG with LASV GP induces tyrosine phosphorylation of β-DG's cytosolic domain as well as it triggers β-DG's dissociation from the cytoskeletal adaptor utrophin [49]. Then, it is envisioned that this later step of detachment of virus-bound DG from the actin-based cytoskeleton may ease subsequent endocytosis of the virus–receptor complex.

2.2. LASV Can Use Phosphatidylserine Receptors to Enter the Cell

The existence of alternative viral receptors was initially suggested by the observations that certain cell-types deficient in functional α-DG, i.e., hepatocytes, could be highly susceptible to LASV infection and that mice lacking the LARGE gene sustain LASV replication at a level comparable to that in wild-type mice [35,50]. cDNA library screening studies from Kawaoka's group singled out the Tyro3/Axl/Mer (TAM) receptor tyrosine kinases Axl and Tyro3/Dtk as potential LASV receptor candidates [51]. TAM family members are tyrosine-kinases which expose tandem immunoglobulin-related domains to the extracellular matrix. These domains interact with host protein S (ProS) and growth arrest-specific gene 6 (Gas6), which are serum proteins that bind the negatively charged phospholipid phosphatidylserine (PtdSer). PtdSer is translocated from the inner leaflet to the external leaflet of the plasma membrane in apoptotic cells, where it acts as a signal for professional phagocytes (macrophages and dendritic cells) as well as non-professional phagocytes (e.g., epithelial cells) [52,53]. TAM receptors have been shown to play a role in virus entry of several RNA viruses such as Ebola (EBOV), dengue (DENV) and Zika, through a mechanism termed "apoptotic mimicry" [54–56]. This mechanism involves recognition of PtdSer exposed on the viral surface, incorporated from the cellular lipid bilayer during the budding process, as a signal for virus uptake [57–59]. Of note, there is evidence that cells infected with the NW arenavirus Pichinde display PtdSer on their plasma membranes; therefore, it is reasonable to conceive that both NW and OW arenaviruses could benefit from PtdSer receptors for viral entry [60]. In the case of LASV, initial studies using a HIV-based lentiviral vector pseudotyped with LASV GP empirically confirmed the capability of Axl to facilitate viral entry to cells lacking optimal carbohydrate modification of α-DG or to DG knockout cells [51]. Experiments from the Choe's group applying alternative lentiviral pseudotyped platforms showed no enhancement of LASV (or LCMV) entry upon overexpression of Axl in human embryonic kidney (HEK-293T) cells [61] and hypothesized that LASV internalization via α-DG may be preferred over PtdSer receptors. Later, experiments from the Kunz's group using a recombinant LCMV system expressing LASV GP (rLCMV-LASVGP) ultimately confirmed that the endogenous expression of Axl does not actually enhance viral entry in the presence of fully functional α-DG receptor but it strongly augments viral infection in the absence of α-DG [62].

In line with these findings, T-cell immunoglobulin mucin I (TIM-1) has also been recently identified as a PtdSer receptor for LASV entry [63]. TIM receptors are cell surface glycoproteins that display an extracellular immunoglobulin variable-like domain (IgV), bearing a structural pocket with high affinity for PtdSer [64]. Unlike TAM receptors, TIM directly binds PtdSer, without the need for the Gas6 or ProS adaptors. It was demonstrated that TIM-I also mediates entry of vesicular stomatitis virus pseudovirions bearing LASV GP, either in the absence of α-DG or under conditions where it is inadequately glycosylated [63]. This behavior resembles that of Axl, suggesting a similarity between the entry route promoted by TAM and TIM receptors. In this sense, although functional α-DG would be the first LASV receptor of choice, the use of PtdSer receptors could function as a non-canonical GP-independent mechanism exploited by the virus to expand the spectrum of cellular tropism.

2.3. *DC-SIGN and LSECtin Lectin Receptors Can Mediate LASV Cell Entry*

Two additional receptor candidates were identified in the cDNA screening studies [51]: dendritic cell-specific intercellular adhesion molecule -3 grabbing nonintegrin (DC-SIGN) and liver and lymph node sinusoidal endothelial calcium-dependent lectin (LSECtin), both of which belong to the calcium-dependent (C-type) family of lectins. Of note, there is previous evidence indicating that DC-SIGN can facilitate infection of the NW JUNV and other enveloped viruses, including EBOV and Rift Valley fever virus [65–67]. Likewise, LSECtin has been implicated in entry of EBOV, SARs coronavirus and Japanese encephalitis virus [68–70]. As observed for TAM receptors, both DC-SIGN and LSECtin enhanced the susceptibility of cells to infection by LASV GP-pseudotyped lentivirus and participate in LASV entry independently of α-DG [51]. These lectin receptors were more effective at enhancing virus infection than TAM receptors, but importantly, none of these alternative receptors showed higher efficiency than properly modified α-DG, the principal portal of entry for LASV [51] (Figure 1). It was also shown that DC-SIGN or LSECtin binding to LASV GP is carbohydrate-specific, a fact that is characteristic of this C-type lectins family [51]. Strikingly, experiments using monocyte-derived immature human dendritic cells (MDDCs), which lack expression of Axl and Tyro3, demonstrated that upregulated expression of DC-SIGN correlates with enhanced virus attachment and productive infection, and that highly mannosylated glycans exposed on LASV GP1 surface interact with DC-SIGN during attachment [71]. Thus, DC-SIGN and LSECtin may facilitate LASV entry into dendritic cells, which represent the preferred early targets for arenavirus infection [72,73].

2.4. *LASV Entry Involves Macropinocytosis and Intracellular LAMP1 Receptor for Virus Fusion*

Upon receptor binding, OW arenaviruses including LASV, enter the host cell by a clathrin-independent endocytic process followed by transport to late endosomal compartments, where pH-dependent fusion of viral and cell membrane takes place [74,75]. Strikingly, sodium hydrogen exchangers (NHEs) have been identified through a genome-wide small interfering RNA screen, as host factors involved in the multiplication of LCMV in human cells [76]. Based on pharmacological and genetic analysis, Iwasaki et al. further validated NHE as entry factors for LCMV and LASV, implicating macropinocytosis in arenavirus entry [77]. Moreover, using the pseudotyped rLCMV-LASVGP and a panel of specific inhibitors for cellular factors involved in the regulation of macropinocytosis, Oppliger et al. showed that DG-mediated LASV entry depends on regulatory factors, including NHE, associated with this pathway [78].

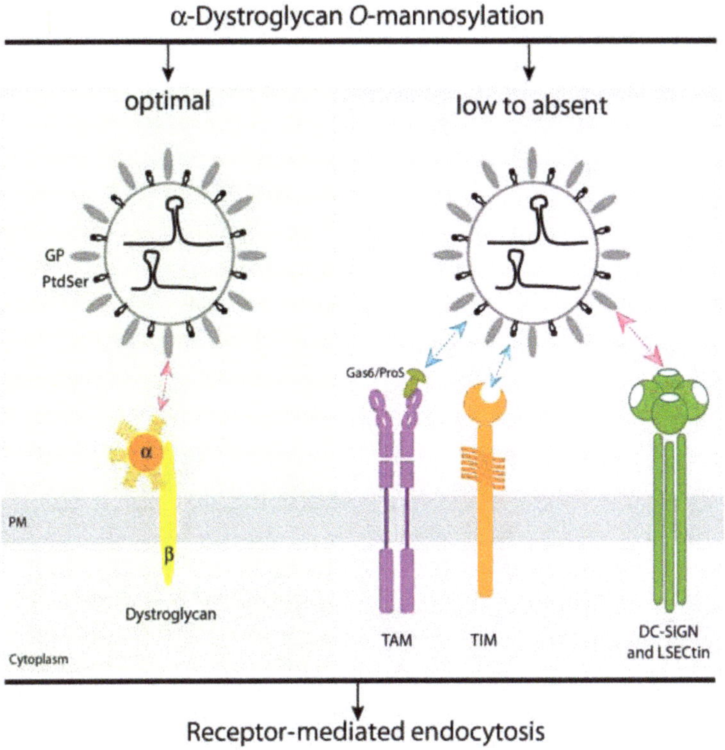

Figure 1. Model of cell receptor/s recognition by Lassa virus (LASV). Left panel. The α-dystroglycan (α-DG) receptor needs to be *O*-mannosylated for efficient virus attachment. In the presence of a fully functional α-DG receptor, LASV enters host cells after binding to the matriglycan platform displayed on α-DG. Right panel. In the absence of α-DG or in conditions where it is inadequately glycosylated, phosphatidylserine (PtdSer)-binding receptors (TAM; TIM) and C-type lectin receptors (DC-SIGN; LSECtin) can mediate α-DG-independent entry. TAM kinases bind Gas6 or ProS serum proteins, which bind to PtdSer molecules exposed on the viral envelope membrane. TIM directly binds PtdSer, without a need for the Gas6 or ProS adaptors. C-type lectins interact with glycans on the LASV glycoprotein (GP). PM: plasma membrane; TAM: Tyro3/Axl/Mer; TIM: T-cell immunoglobulin mucin; DC-SIGN: dendritic cell-specific intercellular adhesion molecule-3 nonintegrin; LSECtin: liver and lymph node sinusoidal endothelial calcium-dependent lectin. Cartoon diagram not to scale.

An unbiased haploid genetic screening in α-DG-deficient cells pinpointed the lysosome-associated membrane protein 1 (LAMP1) as a late endosomal co-receptor specifically required for efficient LASV entry [79]. LAMP1 is mostly found in lysosomes, but it also locates in other endosomal structures. It is hypothesized that the acidic pH of the late endosome destabilizes the high affinity interaction between LASV GP and α-DG, resulting in a "receptor switch" to LAMP1. In this sense, LAMP1 would work as a secondary intracellular receptor that helps induce the GP conformational changes needed for virus fusion. This interpretation is supported by a series of biochemical studies that demonstrated that LAMP1 directly interacts with LASV GP in a pre-fusion configuration, and which described that the strength of this interaction is modulated by pH conditions, where a drop in pH can destabilize LASV GP affinity for α-DG, thereby inducing potent binding to LAMP1 [79]. Furthermore, structural and functional studies showed that LASV GP1 conformation is stable at low pH conditions, at which it displays a triad of histidine residues that are involved in LAMP1 binding [80,81]. In this regard, LAMP1 facilitates LASV exit from earlier endosomal compartments, avoiding prolonged exposure to a harsh proteolytic environment, increasing the overall efficiency of LASV entry and infection [82]. Besides LAMP1, the haploid genetics screening also pointed out α-2,3-sialyltransferase ST3GAL4, as well as additional factors involved in N-glycosylation and sialylation, as being important for LASV entry. Mutations in ST3GAL4, yielding a specific deficiency in sialylation of LAMP1, totally abrogate its ability to interact with LASV GP [79]. This highlights the strict requirement of a specific glycosylated version of LAMP1 for the biochemical interaction with GP to take place. In sum, it is envisioned that LASV would initially attach to the cell surface via α-DG, a step which would lead to delivery of virions to endosomes. Later, as virus-containing vesicles acidify, LASV would dissociate from the α-DG receptor, gaining affinity for LAMP1, and therefore completing the internalization process in a LASV-unique manner that is distinguishable from a standard endocytic process [83,84].

Altogether, these findings describing virus–host interactions involved in LASV entry disclose the diverse spectrum of mechanisms implemented by the virus to efficiently fulfill its internalization and fusion. On the one hand, the ability to utilize entry strategies alternative to α-DG receptor (such as PtdSer or lectin receptors), provides the virion with versatility to enlarge its cell tropism and promotes access to selected cell-targets such as dendritic cells, which are high privileged sites for early LASV productive infection. On the other side, LASV engagement of the late endosomal receptor LAMP1 likely guarantees the optimal spatial conditions required for virus fusion in close proximity to the endosome membrane. Given that not only α-DG- but also Axl-mediated entry involve LAMP1 co-factor [62], it is conceivable that multiple pathways converge at similar late endosomal compartments to efficiently accomplish LASV entry.

3. Role of Virus–Host Interactions Involving the LASV Replication Complex

3.1. Role of DEAD-Box RNA Helicase 3 (DDX3) in Viral Replication

A series of large-scale proteomic studies applying mass-spectrometry have been undertaken to comprehensively identify novel human protein candidates that could interact with the arenavirus proteins [85–89]. Special attention has been paid to NP-binding partners due to the multifunctional role of NP in the viral cycle, which involves crucial interactions with L and Z viral proteins [12,13,15–17,90], and its ability to hijack host factors to inhibit the antiviral innate immune response [19,22,24,91]. It is believed that identifying essential NP–host cell protein interactions can pave the way in the rational design of novel strategies to tackle arenavirus infections. One of the LASV NP interactors recently identified in human cells is DDX3, a protein belonging to the DEAD (Asp-Glu-Ala-Asp) box RNA helicase family, which harbors ATPase and RNA helicase activities [89]. Of note, DDX3 has also emerged in proteomic studies of virus-infected cells, as a novel interacting partner of the OW LCMV and the NW JUNV NPs [85]. CRISPR/Cas9-mediated deletion of DDX3 gene has been shown to lead to a significant reduction in virus yields of LASV, LCMV or JUNV in cell culture. Subsequently, lentiviral-mediated reconstitution of DDX3 expression resulted in a notable recovery in the infection rate of the three viruses, indicating a relevant role of DDX3 in virus growth as a proviral cellular factor [89].

DDX3 is known to be involved in multiple steps of RNA metabolism, including RNA transcription and the initiation of translation in host cells [92–94]. As other DEAD-box RNA helicases, such as DDX1 and DDX5, DDX3 appears to facilitate replication of different RNA viruses, as the alphavirus Venezuelan equine encephalitis virus and the hepatitis C virus (HCV), among others [95–100]. DDX3 is also required for translation of mRNAs containing a long or structured 5′ untranslated region (UTR), such as human immunodeficiency virus type-1 (HIV-1) genomic RNA (gRNA). Indeed, it was reported that DDX3 interacts with the 5′ region of the target mRNA, binds the eukaryotic translation initiation factor 4G (eIF4G) and poly A-binding protein cytoplasmic 1 (PABP), and interacts with HIV-1 Tat protein to facilitate translation of HIV-1 mRNAs [96,101]. In reference to arenaviruses, it was demonstrated that translation of a synthetic arenavirus mRNA analog was unaffected in DDX3-deficient cells, indicating no critical engagement of DDX3 in viral mRNA translation initiation [89]. In contrast, minireplicon assay-based experiments demonstrated that the pro-arenaviral activity of DDX3 strongly depends on DDX3's ability to promote viral RNA synthesis, involving both previously described DDX3 ATPase and helicase RNA-unwinding activities in this function [89,102].

Strikingly, alternative roles have been ascribed to DDX3 in the context of different viral infections [103,104]. On the one hand, DDX3 is considered an antiviral factor given that it is involved in the innate immune response against some viruses such as HIV-1, DENV and HCV [105–107]. DDX3 has been shown to collaborate in the production of IFN-I, through interaction with components of the RIG-I-mediated IFN-I induction pathway [108–110]. However, in contrast to this IFN-I promoting capacity of DDX3, mechanistic analysis has provided evidence that, in the case of LCMV, DDX3 suppresses the IFN-I response at late times of infection, still it remains to be confirmed whether this IFN-I-suppressive role of DDX3 is sustained in the context of an infection with the pathogenic LASV [89]. Secondly, DDX3 is known to be an essential component for stress granule (SG) assembly, and to interact with other SG proteins, such as eIF4E [111]. Different proteomic approaches based on mass-spectrometry have singled out new arenavirus NP-binding candidates related to the SG biology; including but not limited to the Ras GTPase-activating protein-binding protein 1 (G3BP1), eIF2α, apoptosis-inducing factor mitochondrion-associated 1 (AIFM1) and PABP, yet none of them have been confirmed as LASV interactors by alternative biochemical methods [85,89]. Of note, colocalization experiments have revealed the association of the NW arenavirus TCRV replication–transcription complexes (RTCs), where NP accumulates, with G3BP1 and a non-canonical collection of ribosomal proteins, including the ribosomal proteins RPS6 and RPL10a, as well as translation initiation factors eIF4G and eIF4A [112]. In this regard, the finding that JUNV infection inhibits SG formation [113] might be related to the NP-mediated sequestration of DDX3 and other SG-related proteins, resulting in the lack of availability of essential factors needed for SG nucleation. Similarly, in the case of influenza virus infections, it has been hypothesized that the interaction of DDX3 with the viral NS1 protein prevents DDX3 binding to eIF4E and PABP1 as well as DDX3–NP interaction, thus suppressing SG formation, NP recruitment into SGs, and DDX3 antiviral activity [114]. Therefore, it is possible that in a similar way, LASV NP may counteract DDX3 antiviral function and in turn use DDX3 to enhance its own replication.

3.2. Other RNA Helicases Potentially Involved in LASV Replication

In addition to DDX3, a number of cellular proteins functionally related to RNA biosynthesis and ribonucleoprotein complex assembly, including the DEAD-box helicase 5 (DDX5, also referred to as RNA helicase p68) and RNA helicase A (namely DHX9), members of the DExD/Hbox protein family, have been identified as potential overlapping targets of the LCMV L protein and the NP of LASV, LCMV, and/or JUNV (Figure 2) [85,87,89]. Moreover, they have already been confirmed as interactors of the RNA-dependent RNA polymerase (RdRp) of other RNA viruses. For example, DDX5 has been shown to interact with the C-terminal region of HCV NS5B, and has been suggested to be part of the HCV replicase complex [115]. Similarly, DDX5 associates with the influenza A virus PB1 and PB2 proteins [116] and it is needed for an efficient activity of the viral polymerase [117]. Evidence has been provided that DHX9 interacts with the viral genomic RNA and non-structural protein 3 (nsP3) within active replication complexes in Chikungunya virus (CHIKV)-infected cells, displaying an inhibitory effect on viral RNA synthesis and an enhancing effect on viral genome translation, which may imply a regulatory role in CHIKV life cycle [118]. Porcine reproductive and respiratory syndrome virus (family *Arteriviridae*) nucleocapsid protein interacts with DHX9 polymerase to overcome premature termination of viral RNA synthesis [119]. Overall, DExD/H-box helicases emerge as host factors selectively hijacked by polymerases and nucleocapsid or nonstructural proteins from several viruses to facilitate their multiplication. Further work must be carried out to validate the binding of DDX5 and DHX9 helicases to LASV and/or other arenavirus proteins and provide a mechanistic model that could explain the relevance of these interactions.

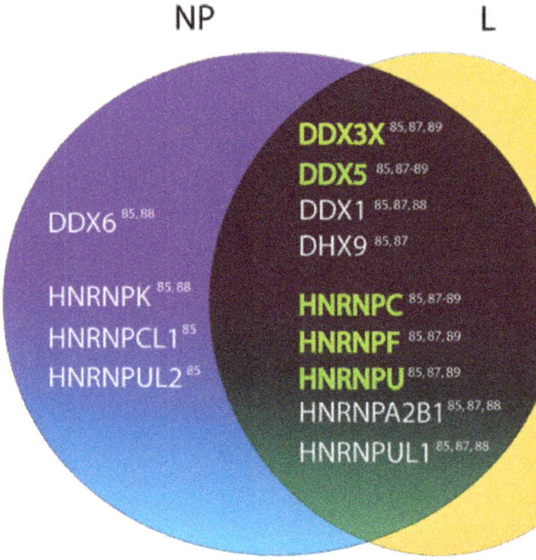

Figure 2. Cellular DExD/H-box helicases and heterogeneous nuclear ribonucleoproteins (hnRNPs) identified among binding partners of the nucleoproteins (NPs) of LASV, lymphocytic choriomeningitis virus (LCMV), and/or Junín virus (JUNV) in different proteomics approaches [85,88,89]. Targets common to the LCMV L polymerase [87] are depicted. LASV NP binding partners are highlighted in green. References are indicated for each target.

Given the observation that many host factors converge as common binding-partners of RNA viruses, it is intriguing whether this is a consequence of the conserved conformational structure shared among proteins from different families of viruses. In particular, segmented negative strand viruses (sNSV) polymerases share key conserved motifs, specifically those corresponding to the fingers, palm and thumb subdomains within the RdRp domain located in the central part of the polypeptide chain. The central ring-like RdRp domain is linked to appendages that would be dedicated to 5′ mRNA capping activities [120–123]. Based on the amino acid sequence motif conservation displayed by sNSV polymerases and the structural similarity between the polymerases of the bunyavirus La Crosse encephalitis virus and influenza virus revealed by crystallographic studies, an overall structural configuration has been proposed for arenavirus L protein. It consists of a canonical RdRp core with N- and C- extensions that form a cavity connected to the exterior by four tunnels (NTP entry, template entry, template exit, and product exit) [124,125]. Structural information has led to a model for sNSV vRNA synthesis in which the L protein would operate in either transcription mode or replication mode, not only during initiation, but also along the whole RNA synthesis process [125,126]. A key question that needs to be addressed is how the polymerase switches from one mode to the other. For arenaviruses, there is genetic and biochemical evidence that L–L interaction is essential for polymerase activity, suggesting that the L polymerase may function in an oligomeric conformation [127]. Thus, as proposed for influenza virus [128,129], a conformational transition of the polymerase from a monomeric state during transcription to an oligomeric state during replication might be hypothesized. In this sense, it is probable that the association with cellular partners may additionally modulate the switch from the transcriptase to the replicase mode of the arenavirus polymerase. To date, DDX3 is the sole NP and L protein interactor for LASV or any other arenavirus that has been demonstrated to contribute in viral RNA synthesis, although the precise underlying mechanism remains to be fully understood. However, it is tempting to speculate that the binding of DDX3 (and eventually other cellular RNA helicases) with NP and L in a replicase complex, may contribute to the unwinding of viral RNA secondary structures such as RNA hairpins within the non-coding intergenic regions, which must be read-through during replication to accomplish full length genome and antigenome RNA synthesis. Likewise, DDX3 and/or other host helicases may facilitate encapsidation of the nascent chain by NP during replication.

3.3. Host Heterogeneous Nuclear Ribonucleoproteins as Candidate Factors Required for the LASV Life Cycle

Other host factors that have recently emerged as potential candidate partners of LASV as well as LCMV and JUNV NP and/or L polymerase are the components of the heterogeneous nuclear ribonucleoprotein (hnRNP) family, including hnRNPA2/B1, one of the most abundant hnRNPs belonging to the A/B type [85,88,89]. HnRNPs are RNA-binding proteins involved in processing pre-mRNAs as well as in mRNA translation, trafficking and stability. Notably, previous reports have already demonstrated the interaction between JUNV NP and hnRNP A1 and that depletion of hnRNP A1 and A2 caused a strong inhibition of virus yield, suggesting a key role of hnRNPs A/B in JUNV multiplication [130]. Additionally, hnRNP K, an LCMV and JUNV NP binding partner detected in the proteomic screening by King et al. [85], has also been reported as a necessary host factor required for JUNV multiplication [131]. Likewise, studies from different groups have similarly ascribed relevant functions to hnRNPs in other viral infections. For example, hnRNP A2/B1 has been proposed to work as a positive regulator in viral RNA synthesis of influenza A virus, hnRNP A2 has been shown to regulate the trafficking of HIV-1 genomic RNA, and hnRNP K has been shown to support vesicular stomatitis virus replication by regulating cell survival and cellular gene expression [132–134]. Altogether, although further research needs to be completed to unveil the importance of hnRNPs in the *Arenaviridae* family, it is intriguing whether any of these proteins would specifically associate with the LASV RNP complex, playing a critical function either in viral genome transcription and/or replication.

3.4. Z Protein Interactors

Arenavirus Z matrix protein has been proposed to drive a mechanism to ensure accurate packaging of all necessary virion components. Apart from its pivotal role in virus assembly and budding [135,136], Z also inhibits viral RNA synthesis by directly binding the L polymerase to trigger its catalytic inactivation, and this can still occur in the absence of host cellular factors [137,138]. Of note, it has been hypothesized that the Z–L complex not only guarantees downregulation of viral gene expression, but also serves as a platform for the functional polymerase to remain locked on the template and be properly packaged into the mature virion [138]. Interestingly, a recent proteomics approach based on JUNV Z has pinpointed a number of targets that were incorporated to Z virus-like particles (VLPs) and purified JUNV particles and which include common interactors of the L and NP proteins, such as DDX3, DDX5, DHX9, hnRNPA2/B1, and PABP [86]. Actually, this is not a totally unexpected observation. For instance, it has been demonstrated for HIV-1 that DHX9 protein stimulates transcription of HIV-1 RNA as well as it associates with the Gag protein to ensure it is adequately recruited into virus particles during the assembly process [139]. In line with this, it is predictable that the association of Z protein with key cellular factors required for viral RNA synthesis may concomitantly facilitate virus packaging and/or make these factors available to complement the activity of viral RNP upon cell entry.

4. Concluding Remarks

LASV is currently considered a top priority emerging pathogen causing severe hemorrhagic fever outbreaks [140]. At this moment, treatment is limited to the nonspecific antiviral ribavirin, shown to be partially effective in LASV infections [141], and the use of favipiravir is still under investigation [142,143]. Moreover, there is no FDA-approved vaccine against LASV or any other arenavirus to date. Therefore, there is an urgent need to develop novel approaches to combat and prevent the infection with these viruses.

In the last years, several reports have provided robust evidence that LASV can utilize alternative entry factors apart from the well-characterized α-DG [144]. Novel lectin and PtdSer receptors have emerged as non-canonical LASV ports of entry, proposed to enhance the viral cell tropism and/or redirect infection to selected cell types.

Studies on virus–host interactions have also improved our understanding of the mechanisms driving LASV replication. A recent series of proteomic approaches oriented to the analysis of the interactome of arenavirus NP, L, and Z proteins in human cells singled out several host factors, such as DExD/H-box helicases and heterogeneous nuclear RNPs, which might be potentially involved in arenavirus RNA synthesis. Particularly, it was demonstrated that the DDX3 ATP-dependent RNA helicase is a LASV target and may be dually exploited to both suppress the host immunity and promote viral replication and/or transcription, since DDX3 ATPase and helicase activities are involved in promoting optimal levels of viral RNA synthesis. Notably, it has recently been reported that a chemical compound directed to an RNA binding site of DDX3 protein displayed broad-spectrum antiviral activity against HIV drug-resistant strains, HCV, DENV, and West Nile virus infection [145]. In this regard, it is intriguing whether the use of DDX3-blocking compounds could be tentatively applied as a novel weapon to battle LASV infections.

Funding: M.E.L., A.D.A. and N.L. are members of the Argentinean Council of Investigation (CONICET). This research received no external funding.

Acknowledgments: The authors would like to apologize to all those researchers whose excellent studies were not included in this review due to space limitations.

Conflicts of Interest: The authors declare no conflict of interest.

References

1. Maes, P.; Alkhovsky, S.V.; Bao, Y.; Beer, M.; Birkhead, M.; Briese, T.; Buchmeier, M.J.; Calisher, C.H.; Charrel, R.N.; Choi, I.R.; et al. Taxonomy of the family Arenaviridae and the order Bunyavirales: Update 2018. *Arch. Virol.* **2018**, *163*, 2295–2310. [CrossRef]
2. Basler, C.F. Molecular pathogenesis of viral hemorrhagic fever. *Semin. Immunopathol.* **2017**, *39*, 551–561. [CrossRef] [PubMed]
3. Ogbu, O.; Ajuluchukwu, E.; Uneke, C.J. Lassa fever in West African sub-region: An overview. *J. Vector Borne Dis.* **2007**, *44*, 1–11. [PubMed]
4. Cashman, K.A.; Wilkinson, E.R.; Zeng, X.; Cardile, A.P.; Facemire, P.R.; Bell, T.M.; Bearss, J.J.; Shaia, C.I.; Schmaljohn, C.S. Immune-Mediated Systemic Vasculitis as the Proposed Cause of Sudden-Onset Sensorineural Hearing Loss following Lassa Virus Exposure in Cynomolgus Macaques. *mBio* **2018**, *9*, e01896-18. [CrossRef] [PubMed]
5. Mateer, E.J.; Huang, C.; Shehu, N.Y.; Paessler, S. Lassa fever-induced sensorineural hearing loss: A neglected public health and social burden. *PLoS Negl. Trop. Dis.* **2018**, *12*, e0006187. [CrossRef]
6. Buchmeier, M.J.; De la Torre, J.C.; Peters, C.J. *Arenaviridae: The Viruses and Their Replication*; Wolters Kluwer Health/Lippincott Williams & Wilkins: Philadelphia, PA, USA, 2007.
7. Kiening, M.; Weber, F.; Frishman, D. Conserved RNA structures in the intergenic regions of ambisense viruses. *Sci. Rep.* **2017**, *7*, 16625. [CrossRef]
8. Eschli, B.; Quirin, K.; Wepf, A.; Weber, J.; Zinkernagel, R.; Hengartner, H. Identification of an N-terminal trimeric coiled-coil core within arenavirus glycoprotein 2 permits assignment to class I viral fusion proteins. *J. Virol.* **2006**, *80*, 5897–5907. [CrossRef]
9. Burri, D.J.; da Palma, J.R.; Kunz, S.; Pasquato, A. Envelope glycoprotein of arenaviruses. *Viruses* **2012**, *4*, 2162–2181. [CrossRef]
10. Hastie, K.M.; Saphire, E.O. Lassa virus glycoprotein: Stopping a moving target. *Curr. Opin. Virol.* **2018**, *31*, 52–58. [CrossRef]
11. Hass, M.; Golnitz, U.; Muller, S.; Becker-Ziaja, B.; Gunther, S. Replicon system for Lassa virus. *J. Virol.* **2004**, *78*, 13793–13803. [CrossRef]
12. Lee, K.J.; Novella, I.S.; Teng, M.N.; Oldstone, M.B.; de La Torre, J.C. NP and L proteins of lymphocytic choriomeningitis virus (LCMV) are sufficient for efficient transcription and replication of LCMV genomic RNA analogs. *J. Virol.* **2000**, *74*, 3470–3477. [CrossRef]

13. Lopez, N.; Jacamo, R.; Franze-Fernandez, M.T. Transcription and RNA replication of tacaribe virus genome and antigenome analogs require N and L proteins: Z protein is an inhibitor of these processes. *J. Virol.* **2001**, *75*, 12241–12251. [CrossRef] [PubMed]
14. Casabona, J.C.; Levingston Macleod, J.M.; Loureiro, M.E.; Gomez, G.A.; Lopez, N. The RING domain and the L79 residue of Z protein are involved in both the rescue of nucleocapsids and the incorporation of glycoproteins into infectious chimeric arenavirus-like particles. *J. Virol.* **2009**, *83*, 7029–7039. [CrossRef]
15. Ortiz-Riano, E.; Cheng, B.Y.; de la Torre, J.C.; Martinez-Sobrido, L. The C-terminal region of lymphocytic choriomeningitis virus nucleoprotein contains distinct and segregable functional domains involved in NP-Z interaction and counteraction of the type I interferon response. *J. Virol.* **2011**, *85*, 13038–13048. [CrossRef] [PubMed]
16. Shtanko, O.; Imai, M.; Goto, H.; Lukashevich, I.S.; Neumann, G.; Watanabe, T.; Kawaoka, Y. A role for the C terminus of Mopeia virus nucleoprotein in its incorporation into Z protein-induced virus-like particles. *J. Virol.* **2010**, *84*, 5415–5422. [CrossRef] [PubMed]
17. Qi, X.; Lan, S.; Wang, W.; Schelde, L.M.; Dong, H.; Wallat, G.D.; Ly, H.; Liang, Y.; Dong, C. Cap binding and immune evasion revealed by Lassa nucleoprotein structure. *Nature* **2010**, *468*, 779–783. [CrossRef] [PubMed]
18. Hastie, K.M.; Liu, T.; Li, S.; King, L.B.; Ngo, N.; Zandonatti, M.A.; Woods, V.L.; de la Torre, J.C., Jr.; Saphire, E.O. Crystal structure of the Lassa virus nucleoprotein-RNA complex reveals a gating mechanism for RNA binding. *Proc. Natl. Acad. Sci. USA* **2011**, *108*, 19365–19370. [CrossRef] [PubMed]
19. Carnec, X.; Baize, S.; Reynard, S.; Diancourt, L.; Caro, V.; Tordo, N.; Bouloy, M. Lassa virus nucleoprotein mutants generated by reverse genetics induce a robust type I interferon response in human dendritic cells and macrophages. *J. Virol.* **2011**, *85*, 12093–12097. [CrossRef]
20. Reynard, S.; Russier, M.; Fizet, A.; Carnec, X.; Baize, S. Exonuclease domain of the Lassa virus nucleoprotein is critical to avoid RIG-I signaling and to inhibit the innate immune response. *J. Virol.* **2014**, *88*, 13923–13927. [CrossRef]
21. Huang, Q.; Shao, J.; Lan, S.; Zhou, Y.; Xing, J.; Dong, C.; Liang, Y.; Ly, H. In vitro and in vivo characterizations of the Pichinde viral NP exoribonuclease function. *J. Virol.* **2015**, *89*, 6595–6607. [CrossRef]
22. Pythoud, C.; Rodrigo, W.W.; Pasqual, G.; Rothenberger, S.; Martinez-Sobrido, L.; de la Torre, J.C.; Kunz, S. Arenavirus nucleoprotein targets interferon regulatory factor-activating kinase IKKepsilon. *J. Virol.* **2012**, *86*, 7728–7738. [CrossRef] [PubMed]
23. Rodrigo, W.W.; Ortiz-Riano, E.; Pythoud, C.; Kunz, S.; de la Torre, J.C.; Martinez-Sobrido, L. Arenavirus nucleoproteins prevent activation of nuclear factor kappa B. *J. Virol.* **2012**, *86*, 8185–8197. [CrossRef] [PubMed]
24. Zhou, S.; Cerny, A.M.; Zacharia, A.; Fitzgerald, K.A.; Kurt-Jones, E.A.; Finberg, R.W. Induction and inhibition of type I interferon responses by distinct components of lymphocytic choriomeningitis virus. *J. Virol.* **2010**, *84*, 9452–9462. [CrossRef] [PubMed]
25. Urata, S.; Yasuda, J. Molecular mechanism of arenavirus assembly and budding. *Viruses* **2012**, *4*, 2049–2079. [CrossRef]
26. Shao, J.; Liang, Y.; Ly, H. Human hemorrhagic Fever causing arenaviruses: Molecular mechanisms contributing to virus virulence and disease pathogenesis. *Pathogens* **2015**, *4*, 283–306. [CrossRef] [PubMed]
27. Hayes, M.; Salvato, M. Arenavirus evasion of host anti-viral responses. *Viruses* **2012**, *4*, 2182–2196. [CrossRef]
28. Fedeli, C.; Moreno, H.; Kunz, S. Novel Insights into Cell Entry of Emerging Human Pathogenic Arenaviruses. *J. Mol. Biol.* **2018**, *430*, 1839–1852. [CrossRef] [PubMed]
29. Cao, W.; Henry, M.D.; Borrow, P.; Yamada, H.; Elder, J.H.; Ravkov, E.V.; Nichol, S.T.; Compans, R.W.; Campbell, K.P.; Oldstone, M.B. Identification of alpha-dystroglycan as a receptor for lymphocytic choriomeningitis virus and Lassa fever virus. *Science* **1998**, *282*, 2079–2081. [CrossRef] [PubMed]
30. Spiropoulou, C.F.; Kunz, S.; Rollin, P.E.; Campbell, K.P.; Oldstone, M.B. New World arenavirus clade C, but not clade A and B viruses, utilizes alpha-dystroglycan as its major receptor. *J. Virol.* **2002**, *76*, 5140–51463. [CrossRef]
31. Acciani, M.; Alston, J.T.; Zhao, G.; Reynolds, H.; Ali, A.M.; Xu, B.; Brindley, M. Mutational analysis of Lassa virus glycoprotein highlights regions required for alpha-dystroglycan utilization. *J. Virol.* **2017**, *91*, e00574-17. [CrossRef]
32. Holt, K.H.; Crosbie, R.H.; Venzke, D.P.; Campbell, K.P. Biosynthesis of dystroglycan: Processing of a precursor propeptide. *FEBS Lett.* **2000**, *468*, 79–83. [CrossRef]

33. Ibraghimov-Beskrovnaya, O.; Ervasti, J.M.; Leveille, C.J.; Slaughter, C.A.; Sernett, S.W.; Campbell, K.P. Primary structure of dystrophin-associated glycoproteins linking dystrophin to the extracellular matrix. *Nature* **1992**, *355*, 696–702. [CrossRef]
34. Ibraghimov-Beskrovnaya, O.; Milatovich, A.; Ozcelik, T.; Yang, B.; Koepnick, K.; Francke, U.; Campbell, K.P. Human dystroglycan: Skeletal muscle cDNA, genomic structure, origin of tissue specific isoforms and chromosomal localization. *Hum. Mol. Genet.* **1993**, *2*, 1651–1657. [CrossRef]
35. Barresi, R.; Campbell, K.P. Dystroglycan: From biosynthesis to pathogenesis of human disease. *J. Cell Sci.* **2006**, *119*, 199–207. [CrossRef] [PubMed]
36. Ervasti, J.M.; Campbell, K.P. A role for the dystrophin-glycoprotein complex as a transmembrane linker between laminin and actin. *J. Cell Biol.* **1993**, *122*, 809–823. [CrossRef] [PubMed]
37. Michele, D.E.; Campbell, K.P. Dystrophin-glycoprotein complex: Post-translational processing and dystroglycan function. *J. Biol. Chem.* **2003**, *278*, 15457–15460. [CrossRef] [PubMed]
38. Ervasti, J.M.; Campbell, K.P. Membrane organization of the dystrophin-glycoprotein complex. *Cell* **1991**, *66*, 1121–1131. [CrossRef]
39. Chung, W.; Campanelli, J.T. WW and EF hand domains of dystrophin-family proteins mediate dystroglycan binding. *Mol. Cell Biol. Res. Commun. MCBRC* **1999**, *2*, 162–171. [CrossRef]
40. Imperiali, M.; Thoma, C.; Pavoni, E.; Brancaccio, A.; Callewaert, N.; Oxenius, A. O Mannosylation of alpha-dystroglycan is essential for lymphocytic choriomeningitis virus receptor function. *J. Virol.* **2005**, *79*, 14297–14308. [CrossRef]
41. Kunz, S.; Rojek, J.M.; Kanagawa, M.; Spiropoulou, C.F.; Barresi, R.; Campbell, K.P.; Oldstone, M.B. Posttranslational modification of alpha-dystroglycan, the cellular receptor for arenaviruses, by the glycosyltransferase LARGE is critical for virus binding. *J. Virol.* **2005**, *79*, 14282–14296. [CrossRef]
42. Yoshida-Moriguchi, T.; Campbell, K.P. Matriglycan: A novel polysaccharide that links dystroglycan to the basement membrane. *Glycobiology* **2015**, *25*, 702–713. [CrossRef] [PubMed]
43. Hastie, K.M.; Igonet, S.; Sullivan, B.M.; Legrand, P.; Zandonatti, M.A.; Robinson, J.E.; Garry, R.F.; Rey, F.A.; Oldstone, M.B.; Saphire, E.O. Crystal structure of the prefusion surface glycoprotein of the prototypic arenavirus LCMV. *Nat. Struct. Mol. Biol.* **2016**, *23*, 513–521. [CrossRef]
44. Hastie, K.M.; Zandonatti, M.A.; Kleinfelter, L.M.; Heinrich, M.L.; Rowland, M.M.; Chandran, K.; Branco, L.M.; Robinson, J.E.; Garry, R.F.; Saphire, E.O. Structural basis for antibody-mediated neutralization of Lassa virus. *Science* **2017**, *356*, 923–928. [CrossRef] [PubMed]
45. Kunz, S.; Rojek, J.M.; Perez, M.; Spiropoulou, C.F.; Oldstone, M.B. Characterization of the interaction of lassa fever virus with its cellular receptor alpha-dystroglycan. *J. Virol.* **2005**, *79*, 5979–5987. [CrossRef] [PubMed]
46. Rojek, J.M.; Spiropoulou, C.F.; Campbell, K.P.; Kunz, S. Old World and clade C New World arenaviruses mimic the molecular mechanism of receptor recognition used by alpha-dystroglycan's host-derived ligands. *J. Virol.* **2007**, *81*, 5685–5695. [CrossRef] [PubMed]
47. Kanagawa, M.; Saito, F.; Kunz, S.; Yoshida-Moriguchi, T.; Barresi, R.; Kobayashi, Y.M.; Muschler, J.; Dumanski, J.P.; Michele, D.E.; Oldstone, M.B.; et al. Molecular recognition by LARGE is essential for expression of functional dystroglycan. *Cell* **2004**, *117*, 953–964. [CrossRef]
48. Hara, Y.; Kanagawa, M.; Kunz, S.; Yoshida-Moriguchi, T.; Satz, J.S.; Kobayashi, Y.M.; Zhu, Z.; Burden, S.J.; Oldstone, M.B.; Campbell, K.P. Like-acetylglucosaminyltransferase (LARGE)-dependent modification of dystroglycan at Thr-317/319 is required for laminin binding and arenavirus infection. *Proc. Natl. Acad. Sci. USA* **2011**, *108*, 17426–17431. [CrossRef]
49. Moraz, M.L.; Pythoud, C.; Turk, R.; Rothenberger, S.; Pasquato, A.; Campbell, K.P.; Kunz, S. Cell entry of Lassa virus induces tyrosine phosphorylation of dystroglycan. *Cell. Microbiol.* **2013**, *15*, 689–700. [CrossRef] [PubMed]
50. Imperiali, M.; Sporri, R.; Hewitt, J.; Oxenius, A. Post-translational modification of {alpha}-dystroglycan is not critical for lymphocytic choriomeningitis virus receptor function in vivo. *J. Gen. Virol.* **2008**, *89*, 2713–2722. [CrossRef]
51. Shimojima, M.; Stroher, U.; Ebihara, H.; Feldmann, H.; Kawaoka, Y. Identification of cell surface molecules involved in dystroglycan-independent Lassa virus cell entry. *J. Virol.* **2012**, *86*, 2067–2078. [CrossRef]
52. Lemke, G.; Rothlin, C.V. Immunobiology of the TAM receptors. *Nat. Rev. Immunol.* **2008**, *8*, 327–336. [CrossRef] [PubMed]

53. Lemke, G. Biology of the TAM receptors. *Cold Spring Harb. Perspect. Biol.* **2013**, *5*, a009076. [CrossRef] [PubMed]
54. Shimojima, M.; Takada, A.; Ebihara, H.; Neumann, G.; Fujioka, K.; Irimura, T.; Jones, S.; Feldmann, H.; Kawaoka, Y. Tyro3 family-mediated cell entry of Ebola and Marburg viruses. *J. Virol.* **2006**, *80*, 10109–10116. [CrossRef] [PubMed]
55. Meertens, L.; Carnec, X.; Lecoin, M.P.; Ramdasi, R.; Guivel-Benhassine, F.; Lew, E.; Lemke, G.; Schwartz, O.; Amara, A. The TIM and TAM families of phosphatidylserine receptors mediate dengue virus entry. *Cell Host Microbe* **2012**, *12*, 544–557. [CrossRef] [PubMed]
56. Meertens, L.; Labeau, A.; Dejarnac, O.; Cipriani, S.; Sinigaglia, L.; Bonnet-Madin, L.; Le Charpentier, T.; Hafirassou, M.L.; Zamborlini, A.; Cao-Lormeau, V.M.; et al. Axl Mediates ZIKA Virus Entry in Human Glial Cells and Modulates Innate Immune Responses. *Cell Rep.* **2017**, *18*, 324–333. [CrossRef] [PubMed]
57. Morizono, K.; Xie, Y.; Olafsen, T.; Lee, B.; Dasgupta, A.; Wu, A.M.; Chen, I.S. The soluble serum protein Gas6 bridges virion envelope phosphatidylserine to the TAM receptor tyrosine kinase Axl to mediate viral entry. *Cell Host Microbe* **2011**, *9*, 286–298. [CrossRef] [PubMed]
58. Mercer, J.; Helenius, A. Vaccinia virus uses macropinocytosis and apoptotic mimicry to enter host cells. *Science* **2008**, *320*, 531–535. [CrossRef]
59. Amara, A.; Mercer, J. Viral apoptotic mimicry. *Nat. Rev. Microbiol.* **2015**, *13*, 461–469. [CrossRef]
60. Soares, M.M.; King, S.W.; Thorpe, P.E. Targeting inside-out phosphatidylserine as a therapeutic strategy for viral diseases. *Nat. Med.* **2008**, *14*, 1357–1362. [CrossRef]
61. Jemielity, S.; Wang, J.J.; Chan, Y.K.; Ahmed, A.A.; Li, W.; Monahan, S.; Bu, X.; Farzan, M.; Freeman, G.J.; Umetsu, D.T.; et al. TIM-family proteins promote infection of multiple enveloped viruses through virion-associated phosphatidylserine. *PLoS Pathog.* **2013**, *9*, e1003232. [CrossRef]
62. Fedeli, C.; Torriani, G.; Galan-Navarro, C.; Moraz, M.L.; Moreno, H.; Gerold, G.; Kunz, S. Axl Can Serve as Entry Factor for Lassa Virus Depending on the Functional Glycosylation of Dystroglycan. *J. Virol.* **2018**, *92*, e01613-17. [CrossRef] [PubMed]
63. Brouillette, R.B.; Phillips, E.K.; Patel, R.; Mahauad-Fernandez, W.; Moller-Tank, S.; Rogers, K.J.; Dillard, J.A.; Cooney, A.L.; Martinez-Sobrido, L.; Okeoma, C.; et al. TIM-1 Mediates Dystroglycan-Independent Entry of Lassa Virus. *J. Virol.* **2018**, *92*, e00093-18. [CrossRef] [PubMed]
64. Freeman, G.J.; Casasnovas, J.M.; Umetsu, D.T.; DeKruyff, R.H. TIM genes: A family of cell surface phosphatidylserine receptors that regulate innate and adaptive immunity. *Immunol. Rev.* **2010**, *235*, 172–189. [CrossRef] [PubMed]
65. Martinez, M.G.; Bialecki, M.A.; Belouzard, S.; Cordo, S.M.; Candurra, N.A.; Whittaker, G.R. Utilization of human DC-SIGN and L-SIGN for entry and infection of host cells by the New World arenavirus, Junin virus. *Biochem. Biophys. Res. Commun.* **2013**, *441*, 612–617. [CrossRef]
66. Leger, P.; Tetard, M.; Youness, B.; Cordes, N.; Rouxel, R.N.; Flamand, M.; Lozach, P.Y. Differential Use of the C-Type Lectins L-SIGN and DC-SIGN for Phlebovirus Endocytosis. *Traffic* **2016**, *17*, 639–656. [CrossRef]
67. Alvarez, C.P.; Lasala, F.; Carrillo, J.; Muniz, O.; Corbi, A.L.; Delgado, R. C-type lectins DC-SIGN and L-SIGN mediate cellular entry by Ebola virus in cis and in trans. *J. Virol.* **2002**, *76*, 6841–6844. [CrossRef]
68. Powlesland, A.S.; Fisch, T.; Taylor, M.E.; Smith, D.F.; Tissot, B.; Dell, A.; Pohlmann, S.; Drickamer, K. A novel mechanism for LSECtin binding to Ebola virus surface glycoprotein through truncated glycans. *J. Biol. Chem.* **2008**, *283*, 593–602. [CrossRef]
69. Gramberg, T.; Hofmann, H.; Moller, P.; Lalor, P.F.; Marzi, A.; Geier, M.; Krumbiegel, M.; Winkler, T.; Kirchhoff, F.; Adams, D.H.; et al. LSECtin interacts with filovirus glycoproteins and the spike protein of SARS coronavirus. *Virology* **2005**, *340*, 224–236. [CrossRef]
70. Shimojima, M.; Takenouchi, A.; Shimoda, H.; Kimura, N.; Maeda, K. Distinct usage of three C-type lectins by Japanese encephalitis virus: DC-SIGN, DC-SIGNR, and LSECtin. *Arch. Virol.* **2014**, *159*, 2023–2031. [CrossRef]
71. Goncalves, A.R.; Moraz, M.L.; Pasquato, A.; Helenius, A.; Lozach, P.Y.; Kunz, S. Role of DC-SIGN in Lassa virus entry into human dendritic cells. *J. Virol.* **2013**, *87*, 11504–11515. [CrossRef]
72. Baize, S.; Kaplon, J.; Faure, C.; Pannetier, D.; Georges-Courbot, M.C.; Deubel, V. Lassa virus infection of human dendritic cells and macrophages is productive but fails to activate cells. *J. Immunol.* **2004**, *172*, 2861–2869. [CrossRef]

73. Macal, M.; Lewis, G.M.; Kunz, S.; Flavell, R.; Harker, J.A.; Zuniga, E.I. Plasmacytoid dendritic cells are productively infected and activated through TLR-7 early after arenavirus infection. *Cell Host Microbe* **2012**, *11*, 617–630. [CrossRef] [PubMed]
74. Quirin, K.; Eschli, B.; Scheu, I.; Poort, L.; Kartenbeck, J.; Helenius, A. Lymphocytic choriomeningitis virus uses a novel endocytic pathway for infectious entry via late endosomes. *Virology* **2008**, *378*, 21–33. [CrossRef] [PubMed]
75. Rojek, J.M.; Sanchez, A.B.; Nguyen, N.T.; de la Torre, J.C.; Kunz, S. Different mechanisms of cell entry by human-pathogenic Old World and New World arenaviruses. *J. Virol.* **2008**, *82*, 7677–7687. [CrossRef] [PubMed]
76. Panda, D.; Das, A.; Dinh, P.X.; Subramaniam, S.; Nayak, D.; Barrows, N.J.; Pearson, J.L.; Thompson, J.; Kelly, D.L.; Ladunga, I.; et al. RNAi screening reveals requirement for host cell secretory pathway in infection by diverse families of negative-strand RNA viruses. *Proc. Natl. Acad. Sci. USA* **2011**, *108*, 19036–19041. [CrossRef] [PubMed]
77. Iwasaki, M.; Ngo, N.; de la Torre, J.C. Sodium hydrogen exchangers contribute to arenavirus cell entry. *J. Virol.* **2014**, *88*, 643–654. [CrossRef]
78. Oppliger, J.; Torriani, G.; Herrador, A.; Kunz, S. Lassa Virus Cell Entry via Dystroglycan Involves an Unusual Pathway of Macropinocytosis. *J. Virol.* **2016**, *90*, 6412–6429. [CrossRef] [PubMed]
79. Jae, L.T.; Raaben, M.; Herbert, A.S.; Kuehne, A.I.; Wirchnianski, A.S.; Soh, T.K.; Stubbs, S.H.; Janssen, H.; Damme, M.; Saftig, P.; et al. Virus entry. Lassa virus entry requires a trigger-induced receptor switch. *Science* **2014**, *344*, 1506–1510. [CrossRef]
80. Cohen-Dvashi, H.; Cohen, N.; Israeli, H.; Diskin, R. Molecular mechanism for LAMP1 recognition by Lassa Virus. *J. Virol.* **2015**, *89*, 7584–7592. [CrossRef]
81. Li, S.; Sun, Z.; Pryce, R.; Parsy, M.L.; Fehling, S.K.; Schlie, K.; Siebert, C.A.; Garten, W.; Bowden, T.A.; Strecker, T.; et al. Acidic pH-Induced conformations and LAMP1 binding of the Lassa Virus glycoprotein spike. *PLoS Pathog.* **2016**, *12*, e1005418. [CrossRef]
82. Hulseberg, C.E.; Fénéant, L.; Szymańska, K.M.; White, J.M. LAMP1 increases the efficiency of Lassa Virus infection by promoting fusion in less acidic endosomal compartments. *MBio* **2018**, *2*, e01818-17. [CrossRef] [PubMed]
83. Cohen-Dvashi, H.; Israeli, H.; Shani, O.; Katz, A.; Diskin, R. Role of LAMP1 Binding and pH Sensing by the Spike Complex of Lassa Virus. *J. Virol.* **2016**, *90*, 10329–10338. [CrossRef] [PubMed]
84. Israeli, H.; Cohen-Dvashi, H.; Shulman, A.; Shimon, A.; Diskin, R. Mapping of the Lassa virus LAMP1 binding site reveals unique determinants not shared by other old world arenaviruses. *PLoS Pathog.* **2017**, *13*, e1006337. [CrossRef] [PubMed]
85. King, B.R.; Hershkowitz, D.; Eisenhauer, P.L.; Weir, M.E.; Ziegler, C.M.; Russo, J.; Bruce, E.A.; Ballif, B.A.; Botten, J. A Map of the Arenavirus Nucleoprotein-Host Protein Interactome Reveals that Junin Virus Selectively Impairs the Antiviral Activity of Double-Stranded RNA-Activated Protein Kinase (PKR). *J. Virol.* **2017**, *91*, e00763-17. [CrossRef] [PubMed]
86. Ziegler, C.M.; Eisenhauer, P.; Kelly, J.A.; Dang, L.N.; Beganovic, V.; Bruce, E.A.; King, B.R.; Shirley, D.J.; Weir, M.E.; Ballif, B.A.; et al. A proteomic survey of Junin virus interactions with human proteins reveals host factors required for arenavirus replication. *J. Virol.* **2018**, *92*, e01565-17. [CrossRef]
87. Khamina, K.; Lercher, A.; Caldera, M.; Schliehe, C.; Vilagos, B.; Sahin, M.; Kosack, L.; Bhattacharya, A.; Majek, P.; Stukalov, A.; et al. Characterization of host proteins interacting with the lymphocytic choriomeningitis virus L protein. *PLoS Pathog.* **2017**, *13*, e1006758. [CrossRef]
88. Iwasaki, M.; Minder, P.; Cai, Y.; Kuhn, J.H.; Yates, J.R., 3rd; Torbett, B.E.; de la Torre, J.C. Interactome analysis of the lymphocytic choriomeningitis virus nucleoprotein in infected cells reveals ATPase Na+/K+ transporting subunit Alpha 1 and prohibitin as host-cell factors involved in the life cycle of mammarenaviruses. *PLoS Pathog.* **2018**, *14*, e1006892. [CrossRef]
89. Loureiro, M.E.; Zorzetto-Fernandes, A.L.; Radoshitzky, S.; Chi, X.; Dallari, S.; Marooki, N.; Leger, P.; Foscaldi, S.; Harjono, V.; Sharma, S.; et al. DDX3 suppresses type I interferons and favors viral replication during Arenavirus infection. *PLoS Pathog.* **2018**, *14*, e1007125. [CrossRef]
90. Loureiro, M.E.; D'Antuono, A.; Levingston Macleod, J.M.; Lopez, N. Uncovering viral protein-protein interactions and their role in arenavirus life cycle. *Viruses* **2012**, *4*, 1651–1667. [CrossRef]

91. Martinez-Sobrido, L.; Zuniga, E.I.; Rosario, D.; Garcia-Sastre, A.; de la Torre, J.C. Inhibition of the type I interferon response by the nucleoprotein of the prototypic arenavirus lymphocytic choriomeningitis virus. *J. Virol.* **2006**, *80*, 9192–9199. [CrossRef]
92. Chang, P.C.; Chi, C.W.; Chau, G.Y.; Li, F.Y.; Tsai, Y.H.; Wu, J.C.; Wu Lee, Y.H. DDX3, a DEAD box RNA helicase, is deregulated in hepatitis virus-associated hepatocellular carcinoma and is involved in cell growth control. *Oncogene* **2006**, *25*, 1991–2003. [CrossRef] [PubMed]
93. Lai, M.C.; Chang, W.C.; Shieh, S.Y.; Tarn, W.Y. DDX3 regulates cell growth through translational control of cyclin E1. *Mol. Cell. Biol.* **2010**, *30*, 5444–5453. [CrossRef]
94. Cruciat, C.M.; Dolde, C.; de Groot, R.E.; Ohkawara, B.; Reinhard, C.; Korswagen, H.C.; Niehrs, C. RNA helicase DDX3 is a regulatory subunit of casein kinase 1 in Wnt-beta-catenin signaling. *Science* **2013**, *339*, 1436–1441. [CrossRef] [PubMed]
95. Ariumi, Y.; Kuroki, M.; Abe, K.; Dansako, H.; Ikeda, M.; Wakita, T.; Kato, N. DDX3 DEAD-box RNA helicase is required for hepatitis C virus RNA replication. *J. Virol.* **2007**, *81*, 13922–13926. [CrossRef]
96. Lai, M.C.; Wang, S.W.; Cheng, L.; Tarn, W.Y.; Tsai, S.J.; Sun, H.S. Human DDX3 interacts with the HIV-1 Tat protein to facilitate viral mRNA translation. *PLoS ONE* **2013**, *8*, e68665. [CrossRef]
97. Yasuda-Inoue, M.; Kuroki, M.; Ariumi, Y. Distinct DDX DEAD-box RNA helicases cooperate to modulate the HIV-1 Rev function. *Biochem. Biophys. Res. Commun.* **2013**, *434*, 803–808. [CrossRef]
98. Chahar, H.S.; Chen, S.; Manjunath, N. P-body components LSM1, GW182, DDX3, DDX6 and XRN1 are recruited to WNV replication sites and positively regulate viral replication. *Virology* **2013**, *436*, 1–7. [CrossRef]
99. Amaya, M.; Brooks-Faulconer, T.; Lark, T.; Keck, F.; Bailey, C.; Raman, V.; Narayanan, A. Venezuelan equine encephalitis virus non-structural protein 3 (nsP3) interacts with RNA helicases DDX1 and DDX3 in infected cells. *Antivir. Res.* **2016**, *131*, 49–60. [CrossRef] [PubMed]
100. Shih, J.W.; Tsai, T.Y.; Chao, C.H.; Wu Lee, Y.H. Candidate tumor suppressor DDX3 RNA helicase specifically represses cap-dependent translation by acting as an eIF4E inhibitory protein. *Oncogene* **2008**, *27*, 700–714. [CrossRef]
101. Soto-Rifo, R.; Rubilar, P.S.; Limousin, T.; de Breyne, S.; Decimo, D.; Ohlmann, T. DEAD-box protein DDX3 associates with eIF4F to promote translation of selected mRNAs. *EMBO J.* **2012**, *31*, 3745–3756. [CrossRef] [PubMed]
102. Garbelli, A.; Beermann, S.; Di Cicco, G.; Dietrich, U.; Maga, G. A motif unique to the human DEAD-box protein DDX3 is important for nucleic acid binding, ATP hydrolysis, RNA/DNA unwinding and HIV-1 replication. *PLoS ONE* **2011**, *6*, e19810. [CrossRef]
103. Ariumi, Y. Multiple functions of DDX3 RNA helicase in gene regulation, tumorigenesis, and viral infection. *Front. Genet.* **2014**, *5*, 423. [CrossRef] [PubMed]
104. Valiente-Echeverria, F.; Hermoso, M.A.; Soto-Rifo, R. RNA helicase DDX3: At the crossroad of viral replication and antiviral immunity. *Rev. Med. Virol.* **2015**, *25*, 286–299. [CrossRef] [PubMed]
105. Gringhuis, S.I.; Hertoghs, N.; Kaptein, T.M.; Zijlstra-Willems, E.M.; Sarrami-Forooshani, R.; Sprokholt, J.K.; van Teijlingen, N.H.; Kootstra, N.A.; Booiman, T.; van Dort, K.A.; et al. HIV-1 blocks the signaling adaptor MAVS to evade antiviral host defense after sensing of abortive HIV-1 RNA by the host helicase DDX3. *Nat. Immunol.* **2017**, *18*, 225–235. [CrossRef]
106. Li, G.; Feng, T.; Pan, W.; Shi, X.; Dai, J. DEAD-box RNA helicase DDX3X inhibits DENV replication via regulating type one interferon pathway. *Biochem. Biophys. Res. Commun.* **2015**, *456*, 327–332. [CrossRef] [PubMed]
107. Oshiumi, H.; Ikeda, M.; Matsumoto, M.; Watanabe, A.; Takeuchi, O.; Akira, S.; Kato, N.; Shimotohno, K.; Seya, T. Hepatitis C virus core protein abrogates the DDX3 function that enhances IPS-1-mediated IFN-beta induction. *PLoS ONE* **2010**, *5*, e14258. [CrossRef] [PubMed]
108. Schroder, M.; Baran, M.; Bowie, A.G. Viral targeting of DEAD box protein 3 reveals its role in TBK1/IKKepsilon-mediated IRF activation. *EMBO J.* **2008**, *27*, 2147–2157. [CrossRef]
109. Soulat, D.; Burckstummer, T.; Westermayer, S.; Goncalves, A.; Bauch, A.; Stefanovic, A.; Hantschel, O.; Bennett, K.L.; Decker, T.; Superti-Furga, G. The DEAD-box helicase DDX3X is a critical component of the TANK-binding kinase 1-dependent innate immune response. *EMBO J.* **2008**, *27*, 2135–2146. [CrossRef] [PubMed]
110. Gu, L.; Fullam, A.; Brennan, R.; Schroder, M. Human DEAD box helicase 3 couples IkappaB kinase epsilon to interferon regulatory factor 3 activation. *Mol. Cell. Biol.* **2013**, *33*, 2004–2015. [CrossRef]

111. Shih, J.W.; Wang, W.T.; Tsai, T.Y.; Kuo, C.Y.; Li, H.K.; Wu Lee, Y.H. Critical roles of RNA helicase DDX3 and its interactions with eIF4E/PABP1 in stress granule assembly and stress response. *Biochem. J.* **2012**, *441*, 119–129. [CrossRef]
112. Baird, N.L.; York, J.; Nunberg, J.H. Arenavirus infection induces discrete cytosolic structures for RNA replication. *J. Virol.* **2012**, *86*, 11301–11310. [CrossRef]
113. Linero, F.N.; Thomas, M.G.; Boccaccio, G.L.; Scolaro, L.A. Junin virus infection impairs stress-granule formation in Vero cells treated with arsenite via inhibition of eIF2alpha phosphorylation. *J. Gen. Virol.* **2011**, *92*, 2889–2899. [CrossRef] [PubMed]
114. Thulasi Raman, S.N.; Liu, G.; Pyo, H.M.; Cui, Y.C.; Xu, F.; Ayalew, L.E.; Tikoo, S.K.; Zhou, Y. DDX3 Interacts with Influenza A Virus NS1 and NP Proteins and Exerts Antiviral Function through Regulation of Stress Granule Formation. *J. Virol.* **2016**, *90*, 3661–3675. [CrossRef] [PubMed]
115. Goh, P.Y.; Tan, Y.J.; Lim, S.P.; Tan, Y.H.; Lim, S.G.; Fuller-Pace, F.; Hong, W. Cellular RNA helicase p68 relocalization and interaction with the hepatitis C virus (HCV) NS5B protein and the potential role of p68 in HCV RNA replication. *J. Virol.* **2004**, *78*, 5288–5298. [CrossRef] [PubMed]
116. Jorba, N.; Juarez, S.; Torreira, E.; Gastaminza, P.; Zamarreno, N.; Albar, J.P.; Ortin, J. Analysis of the interaction of influenza virus polymerase complex with human cell factors. *Proteomics* **2008**, *8*, 2077–2088. [CrossRef]
117. Bortz, E.; Westera, L.; Maamary, J.; Steel, J.; Albrecht, R.A.; Manicassamy, B.; Chase, G.; Martinez-Sobrido, L.; Schwemmle, M.; Garcia-Sastre, A. Host- and strain-specific regulation of influenza virus polymerase activity by interacting cellular proteins. *mBio* **2011**, *16*, e00151-11. [CrossRef] [PubMed]
118. Matkovic, R.; Bernard, E.; Fontanel, S.; Eldin, P.; Chazal, N.; Hassan Hersi, D.; Merits, A.; Peloponese, J.M., Jr.; Briant, L. The host DHX9 DExH Box helicase is recruited to Chikungunya virus replication complexes for optimal genomic RNA translation. *J. Virol.* **2018**, JVI.01764. [CrossRef]
119. Liu, L.; Tian, J.; Nan, H.; Tian, M.; Li, Y.; Xu, X.; Huang, B.; Zhou, E.; Hiscox, J.A.; Chen, H. Porcine Reproductive and Respiratory Syndrome Virus Nucleocapsid Protein Interacts with Nsp9 and Cellular DHX9 To Regulate Viral RNA Synthesis. *J. Virol.* **2016**, *90*, 5384–5398. [CrossRef]
120. Wilda, M.; Lopez, N.; Casabona, J.C.; Franze-Fernandez, M.T. Mapping of the tacaribe arenavirus Z-protein binding sites on the L protein identified both amino acids within the putative polymerase domain and a region at the N terminus of L that are critically involved in binding. *J. Virol.* **2008**, *82*, 11454–11460. [CrossRef]
121. Kranzusch, P.J.; Schenk, A.D.; Rahmeh, A.A.; Radoshitzky, S.R.; Bavari, S.; Walz, T.; Whelan, S.P. Assembly of a functional Machupo virus polymerase complex. *Proc. Natl. Acad. Sci. USA* **2010**, *107*, 20069–20074. [CrossRef]
122. Morin, B.; Coutard, B.; Lelke, M.; Ferron, F.; Kerber, R.; Jamal, S.; Frangeul, A.; Baronti, C.; Charrel, R.; de Lamballerie, X.; et al. The N-terminal domain of the arenavirus L protein is an RNA endonuclease essential in mRNA transcription. *PLoS Pathog.* **2010**, *6*, e1001038. [CrossRef] [PubMed]
123. Brunotte, L.; Lelke, M.; Hass, M.; Kleinsteuber, K.; Becker-Ziaja, B.; Gunther, S. Domain structure of Lassa virus L protein. *J. Virol.* **2011**, *85*, 324–333. [CrossRef] [PubMed]
124. Reguera, J.; Gerlach, P.; Cusack, S. Towards a structural understanding of RNA synthesis by negative strand RNA viral polymerases. *Curr. Opin. Struct. Biol.* **2016**, *36*, 75–84. [CrossRef] [PubMed]
125. Ferron, F.; Weber, F.; de la Torre, J.C.; Reguera, J. Transcription and replication mechanisms of Bunyaviridae and Arenaviridae L proteins. *Virus Res.* **2017**, *234*, 118–134. [CrossRef]
126. Gerlach, P.; Malet, H.; Cusack, S.; Reguera, J. Structural Insights into Bunyavirus Replication and Its Regulation by the vRNA Promoter. *Cell* **2015**, *161*, 1267–1279. [CrossRef]
127. Sanchez, A.B.; de la Torre, J.C. Genetic and biochemical evidence for an oligomeric structure of the functional L polymerase of the prototypic arenavirus lymphocytic choriomeningitis virus. *J. Virol.* **2005**, *79*, 7262–7268. [CrossRef]
128. Chang, S.; Sun, D.; Liang, H.; Wang, J.; Li, J.; Guo, L.; Wang, X.; Guan, C.; Boruah, B.M.; Yuan, L.; et al. Cryo-EM structure of influenza virus RNA polymerase complex at 4.3 A resolution. *Mol. Cell* **2015**, *57*, 925–935. [CrossRef]
129. Ortin, J.; Martin-Benito, J. The RNA synthesis machinery of negative-stranded RNA viruses. *Virology* **2015**, *479–480*, 532–544. [CrossRef]
130. Maeto, C.A.; Knott, M.E.; Linero, F.N.; Ellenberg, P.C.; Scolaro, L.A.; Castilla, V. Differential effect of acute and persistent Junin virus infections on the nucleo-cytoplasmic trafficking and expression of heterogeneous nuclear ribonucleoproteins type A and B. *J. Gen. Virol.* **2011**, *92*, 2181–2190. [CrossRef]

131. Brunetti, J.E.; Scolaro, L.A.; Castilla, V. The heterogeneous nuclear ribonucleoprotein K (hnRNP K) is a host factor required for dengue virus and Junin virus multiplication. *Virus Res.* **2015**, *203*, 84–91. [CrossRef]
132. Chang, C.K.; Chen, C.J.; Wu, C.C.; Chen, S.W.; Shih, S.R.; Kuo, R.L. Cellular hnRNP A2/B1 interacts with the NP of influenza A virus and impacts viral replication. *PLoS ONE* **2017**, *12*, e0188214. [CrossRef] [PubMed]
133. Levesque, K.; Halvorsen, M.; Abrahamyan, L.; Chatel-Chaix, L.; Poupon, V.; Gordon, H.; DesGroseillers, L.; Gatignol, A.; Mouland, A.J. Trafficking of HIV-1 RNA is mediated by heterogeneous nuclear ribonucleoprotein A2 expression and impacts on viral assembly. *Traffic* **2006**, *7*, 1177–1193. [CrossRef] [PubMed]
134. Dinh, P.X.; Das, A.; Franco, R.; Pattnaik, A.K. Heterogeneous nuclear ribonucleoprotein K supports vesicular stomatitis virus replication by regulating cell survival and cellular gene expression. *J. Virol.* **2013**, *87*, 10059–10069. [CrossRef] [PubMed]
135. Strecker, T.; Eichler, R.; Meulen, J.; Weissenhorn, W.; Dieter Klenk, H.; Garten, W.; Lenz, O. Lassa virus Z protein is a matrix protein and sufficient for the release of virus-like particles [corrected]. *J. Virol.* **2003**, *77*, 10700–10705. [CrossRef] [PubMed]
136. Fehling, S.K.; Lennartz, F.; Strecker, T. Multifunctional nature of the arenavirus RING finger protein Z. *Viruses* **2012**, *4*, 2973–3011. [CrossRef] [PubMed]
137. Loureiro, M.E.; Wilda, M.; Levingston Macleod, J.M.; D'Antuono, A.; Foscaldi, S.; Marino Buslje, C.; Lopez, N. Molecular determinants of arenavirus Z protein homo-oligomerization and L polymerase binding. *J. Virol.* **2011**, *85*, 12304–12314. [CrossRef] [PubMed]
138. Kranzusch, P.J.; Whelan, S.P. Arenavirus Z protein controls viral RNA synthesis by locking a polymerase-promoter complex. *Proc. Natl. Acad. Sci. USA* **2011**, *108*, 19743–19748. [CrossRef]
139. Roy, B.B.; Hu, J.; Guo, X.; Russell, R.S.; Guo, F.; Kleiman, L.; Liang, C. Association of RNA helicase a with human immunodeficiency virus type 1 particles. *J. Biol. Chem.* **2006**, *281*, 12625–12635. [CrossRef]
140. WHO. List of Blueprint Priority Diseases. Available online: https://www.who.int/blueprint/priority-diseases/en/ (accessed on 28 January 2019).
141. McCormick, J.B.; King, I.J.; Webb, P.A.; Scribner, C.L.; Craven, R.B.; Johnson, K.M.; Elliott, L.H.; Belmont-Williams, R. Lassa fever. Effective therapy with ribavirin. *N. Engl. J. Med.* **1986**, *314*, 20–26. [CrossRef]
142. Safronetz, D.; Rosenke, K.; Westover, J.B.; Martellaro, C.; Okumura, A.; Furuta, Y.; Geisbert, J.; Saturday, G.; Komeno, T.; Geisbert, T.W.; et al. The broad-spectrum antiviral favipiravir protects guinea pigs from lethal Lassa virus infection post-disease onset. *Sci. Rep.* **2015**, *12*, 14775. [CrossRef]
143. Raabe, V.N.; Kann, G.; Ribner, B.S.; Morales, A.; Varkey, J.B.; Mehta, A.K.; Lyon, G.M.; Vanairsdale, S.; Faber, K.; Becker, S.; et al. Favipiravir and Ribavirin Treatment of Epidemiologically Linked Cases of Lassa Fever. *Clin. Infect. Dis.* **2017**, *1*, 855–859. [CrossRef] [PubMed]
144. Torriani, G.; Galan-Navarro, C.; Kunz, S. Lassa Virus Cell Entry Reveals New Aspects of Virus-Host Cell Interaction. *J. Virol.* **2017**, *91*, 1–8. [CrossRef] [PubMed]
145. Brai, A.; Fazi, R.; Tintori, C.; Zamperini, C.; Bugli, F.; Sanguinetti, M.; Stigliano, E.; Este, J.; Badia, R.; Franco, S.; et al. Human DDX3 protein is a valuable target to develop broad spectrum antiviral agents. *Proc. Natl. Acad. Sci. USA* **2016**, *113*, 5388–5393. [CrossRef] [PubMed]

pathogens

MDPI

Article

Identification of Residues in Lassa Virus Glycoprotein Subunit 2 That Are Critical for Protein Function

Katherine A. Willard [1,†], Jacob T. Alston [1,†], Marissa Acciani [1] and Melinda A. Brindley [2,*]

1 Department of Infectious Diseases, College of Veterinary Medicine, University of Georgia, Athens, GA 30602, USA; kwillard@uga.edu (K.A.W.); jacob.t.alston@gmail.com (J.T.A.); marissa.acciani@uga.edu (M.A.)

2 Department of Infectious Diseases, Department of Population Health, Center for Vaccines and Immunology, College of Veterinary Medicine, University of Georgia, Athens, GA 30602, USA

* Correspondence: mbrindle@uga.edu; Tel.: +1-706-542-5796

† These authors contributed equally to this work.

Received: 28 November 2018; Accepted: 22 December 2018; Published: 26 December 2018

Abstract: Lassa virus (LASV) is an Old World arenavirus, endemic to West Africa, capable of causing hemorrhagic fever. Currently, there are no approved vaccines or effective antivirals for LASV. However, thorough understanding of the LASV glycoprotein and entry into host cells could accelerate therapeutic design. LASV entry is a two-step process involving the viral glycoprotein (GP). First, the GP subunit 1 (GP1) binds to the cell surface receptor and the viral particle is engulfed into an endosome. Next, the drop in pH triggers GP rearrangements, which ultimately leads to the GP subunit 2 (GP2) forming a six-helix-bundle (6HB). The process of GP2 forming 6HB fuses the lysosomal membrane with the LASV envelope, allowing the LASV genome to enter the host cell. The aim of this study was to identify residues in GP2 that are crucial for LASV entry. To achieve this, we performed alanine scanning mutagenesis on GP2 residues. We tested these mutant GPs for efficient GP1-GP2 cleavage, cell-to-cell membrane fusion, and transduction into cells expressing α-dystroglycan and secondary LASV receptors. In total, we identified seven GP2 mutants that were cleaved efficiently but were unable to effectively transduce cells: GP-L280A, GP-L285A/I286A, GP-I323A, GP-L394A, GP-I403A, GP-L415A, and GP-R422A. Therefore, the data suggest these residues are critical for GP2 function in LASV entry.

Keywords: Lassa virus; arenavirus; viral glycoprotein; viral entry; viral fusion; fusion protein

1. Introduction

Mammalian arenaviruses are divided into two subgroups based on geographic distribution: Old World and New World [1]. Both subgroups contain human pathogens capable of causing severe hemorrhagic fever with high morbidity and mortality. Lassa virus (LASV), the pathogen that causes Lassa fever, is an Old World arenavirus endemic to West Africa. Each year, LASV infects several hundred-thousand people resulting in nearly 5000 deaths [2,3]. The 2018 outbreak in Nigeria was more extensive and had a higher case fatality rate (CFR) than normally recorded (CFR of confirmed cases was approximately 25% as of July 2018) [4], which exemplifies the need to develop LASV antivirals and vaccines. Human infections predominantly occur through zoonotic spread from the rodent host *Mastomys natalensis*, and potentially *Hylomyscus pamfi* and *Mastomys erythroleucus* [5,6]. Transmission can occur through direct contact with infected rodent hosts or exposure to rodent excreta/blood. In addition, person-to-person spread can occur through contact with infectious bodily fluids, putting healthcare workers at higher risk [7,8]. Due to the lack of vaccines and effective therapeutics, LASV is categorized as a class A pathogen [9].

The arenavirus particle consists of a host cell-derived lipid envelope encasing a bi-segmented RNA genome in an ambisense orientation. The envelope contains mature trimeric viral glycoprotein

(GP) spikes that are responsible for attachment and entry into the host cell. The glycoprotein precursor (GPC) is produced as a type I membrane protein and is processed twice by host cell peptidases. First, a cellular peptidase in the endoplasmic reticulum (ER) cleaves the stable signal peptide (SSP) subunit from the precursor. Second, subtilisin kexin isozyme-1/site-1 protease (SKI-1/S1P) in the cis-Golgi cleaves GP1 from GP2 [10–12]. The arenavirus signal peptide is not degraded; instead, it becomes part of the trimeric glycoprotein complex serving as a chaperone assisting with protein processing, trafficking, and pH sensing [13–16]. The GP1 and GP2 subunits mediate receptor interactions and membrane fusion, respectively [17–21].

To enter the host cell, enveloped viruses must mediate fusion between the viral envelope and cellular membrane. The arenavirus glycoprotein contains two heptad repeat (HR) domains and an amino-terminal fusion peptide (N-FP) [22], characteristic of class I fusion proteins [19,20], and similar to those of retroviruses, filoviruses, paramyxoviruses, and influenza [17]. Unlike typical class I fusion proteins, the arenavirus GP2 also contains an internal fusion loop (I-FP), which helps mediate fusion [23,24]. Under low-pH, the arenavirus glycoprotein undergoes major conformational changes prior to initiating viral fusion [25]. Interaction between GP1 and lysosomal associated membrane protein 1 (LAMP1) dissociates GP1 from the trimer, activating the GP2 fusion protein [26,27]. During GP2 rearrangement, the fusion peptide/loop inserts into the host membrane. Once multiple GP2 subunits are triggered, the glycoproteins collapse into an energetically favorable conformation known as a six-helix bundle (6HB) [19]. Full collapse of the glycoprotein complex forms a fusion pore, which enables genome release into the cytoplasm [28].

The pre-fusion LASV GP and post-fusion GP2 of lymphocytic choriomeningitis virus (LCMV), a closely related Old World arenavirus, have been crystalized [19,29]. These two structures illustrate the major GP2 conformational changes that occur during fusion. Previous studies on arenavirus GP2 subunits have characterized both the C-terminal domain, required for interactions with SSP, and hydrophobic amino acids within the fusion peptide and fusion loop [23,30]. However, there has not been an extensive characterization of the GP2 subunit as a whole. Therefore, we produced a panel of GP mutants using either insertional or alanine-scanning mutagenesis and functionally characterized them to identify conserved residues that are critical for the fusion process. We identified several residues, that when changed to alanine, did not affect protein processing but inhibited GP2-mediated-fusion, suggesting these residues may be important for GP2 structural rearrangement or lipid interactions.

2. Results

To identify critical residues in LASV GP2, we produced a panel of mutants. This panel included four hemagglutinin (HA) constructs in which the HA epitope tag was inserted at specific locations within GP2. It also included twenty-nine constructs in which conserved charged amino acids were changed to alanine; in two of these constructs, tandem charged residues were mutated together. Finally, we made twenty-six constructs in which hydrophobic amino acids were changed to alanine, which again included two constructs with tandem hydrophobic residues mutated in a single construct.

2.1. Insertional Mutagenesis

The prefusion structure of LASV GP1-GP2 is compact, with the GP2 alpha helices stacked under the GP1 subunit [29]. Although the likelihood of inserting a peptide tag without disturbing the structure and function was low, we added HA peptides at two locations in the ectodomain. The first was inserted after position 303, which we predicted would fill the center core of the structure. The second was inserted after position 375, which added an HA peptide at the tip of the T-loop, close to the membrane in a surface exposed region (Figure 1A). We also added HA peptides to the cytoplasmic tail. One HA peptide was added at the C-terminus (residue 491), a position that is known to tolerate FLAG tag additions. An HA tag was also engineered after residue 487, to maintain the charged residues at the C-terminus. To characterize these HA mutants, we first assessed whether they were efficiently expressed on the cell surface and cleaved by SKI-1/S1P, releasing GP2. Only GP_{FLAG}-491-HA was processed at levels comparable to parental GP_{FLAG} (Figure 1B,D). All of the remaining HA mutants had low (<50%) GP2 production levels compared to parental GP_{FLAG} (Table 1). Incubating cells expressing LASV GP with a low-pH buffer mimics the lysosomal low-pH environment and triggers GP fusion, resulting in robust syncytia formation [31]. Fusion efficiency is determined by comparing the extent of syncytia formation caused by the mutant GP to parental GP. Production of parental GP_{FLAG} protein induced extensive fusion that resulted in large syncytia after low-pH treatment. GP_{FLAG}-491-HA was the only HA construct that induced fusion similarly to parental GP_{FLAG} (Figure 1C,D) as expected based on the surface levels. Taken together, these results suggest that the addition of the HA tag at these locations prevents efficient GP production and processing.

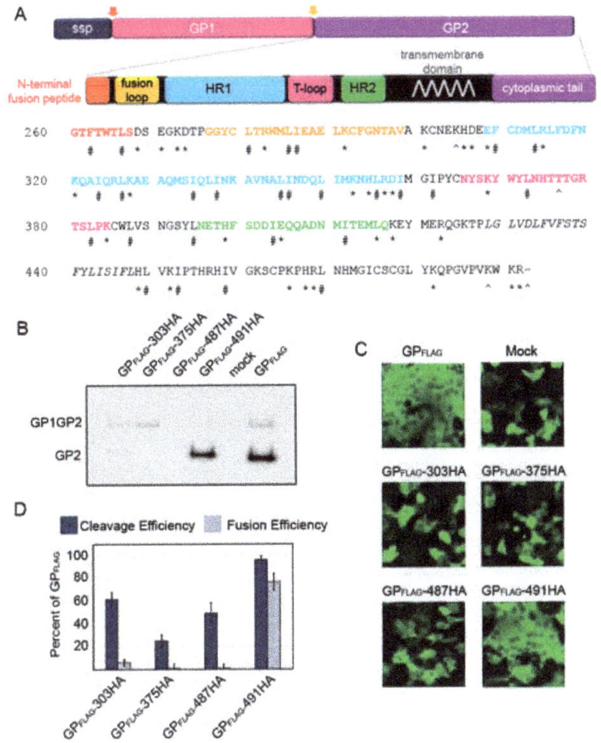

Figure 1. Functional analysis of LASV GP2 HA mutants. (**a**) Schematic of LASV GPC and amino acid sequence of GP2. The signal peptidase cleaves the SSP (red arrow) whereas SKI/S1P cleaves GP1-GP2 (yellow arrow). The known GP2 domains have been color coded, N-terminal fusion peptide (red); internal fusion loop (orange); heptad repeat 1 (blue); the T-loop (magenta); heptad repeat 2 (green); and the transmembrane domain is in italics (grey). The HA tags were inserted before the amino acids labeled with a ^, * denote charged, and # hydrophobic amino acids examined with alanine scanning. (**b**) Representative image of surface biotinylation to assess LASV glycoprotein processing to form GP2. GP1GP2 is the uncleaved glycoprotein precursor. LASV GP_{FLAG} was detected with an anti-FLAG antibody, M2, against the C-terminal GP2 3x FLAG tag. (**c**) Representative images of HA mutants in the cell-to-cell fusion assay. GP_{FLAG} is the parental LASV glycoprotein and mock represents cells transfected with only GFP (no glycoprotein). (**d**) LASV GP2 HA mutant cleavage and fusion efficiencies compared to parental GP_{FLAG}. Error bars represent the standard error of the mean (SEM) from at least three independent trials.

Table 1. Summary of Fusion and GP cleavage of HA mutants.

Mutant	GP2 Protein Expression [1]	Cleavage Efficiency [1]	Fusion Activity [1]
303-HA	14.3 ± 3.5	62.8 ± 6.1	6 ± 2.6
375-HA	1.1 ± 0.1	25.4 ± 5.6	0 ± 3.6
487-HA	1.6 ± 0.4	50.2 ± 9.1	0 ± 3.2
491-HA	55.0 ± 16.1	98.5 ± 3.5	76.3 ± 7.1

[1] All values are displayed as percentage of GP_{FLAG} control ± SEM.

2.2. *Characterization of Charged Constructs*

In order to define individual residues important for GP2 refolding, we made more subtle mutations with alanine scanning mutagenesis. Since charged amino acids are important for protein organization and function [32], we began by mutating 29 highly conserved charged amino acid residues throughout the fusion-active subunit of LASV. We expressed the 29 constructs in Vero cells and monitored the levels of GP present on the cell surface to determine the production and cleavage efficiencies of the constructs (Figure 2A). All mutant glycoproteins except for GP-E308A and GP-H467A/R468A were cleaved producing GP2. GP-H467A/R468A did not produce detectable GP1GP2 or GP2, suggesting this mutation prevents proper protein folding and induced degradation. In contrast, GP-E308A produced a bright GP1GP2 band, which was not cleaved into GP2, indicating that GP1GP2 was produced and trafficked to the surface, but was not cleaved by SKI/S1P (Figure 2A, Table 2).

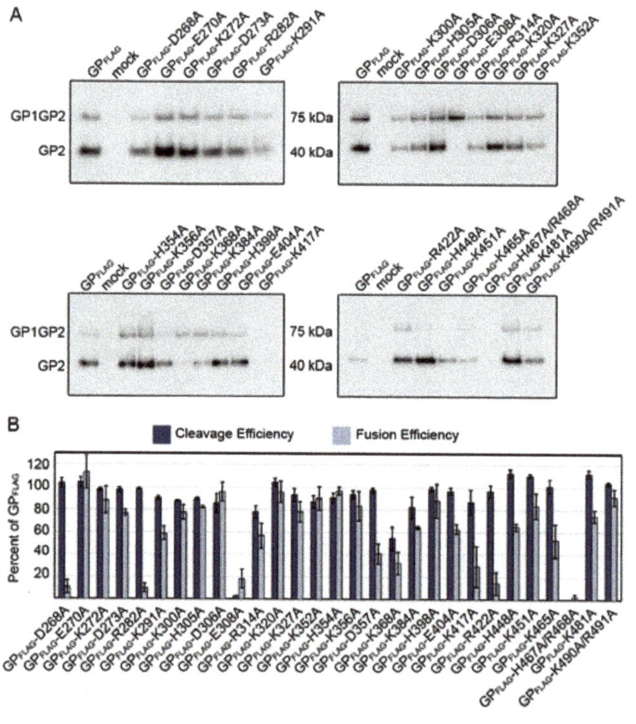

Figure 2. Functional analysis of charged residues in GP2. (**a**) Cell surface proteins were cross-linked to biotin and purified with streptavidin beads. Purified proteins were separated on SDS-PAGE and probed with an anti-FLAG antibody to detect GP, representative immunoblots are shown. (**b**) LASV GP2 mutant cleavage and fusion efficiencies compared to parental GP_{FLAG}. Error bars represent the SEM from at least three independent trials.

Table 2. Summary of GP2 Expression, GP Cleavage, Cell-to-cell Fusion, and Transduction Data.

Mutant [1]	Mutant Type [2]	GP2 Protein Expression [3]	Cleavage Efficiency [3]	Fusion Activity [3]	Transduction Efficiency [3]	
					HAP1	HAP1-ΔDAG
F262A	H	198.3 ± 62.5	108.8 ± 3.1	88.9 ± 6.4	87.2 ± 5.2	94.7 ± 9.3
L266A	H	56.2 ± 6.7	96.3 ± 3.2	81.1 ± 8.4	71.5 ± 8.5	67.7 ± 11.4
D268A	***C***	***118.6 ± 46.2***	***103.4 ± 4.2***	***10.8 ± 5.0***	***94.1 ± 1.8***	***86.0 ± 5.5***
E270A	C	187.4 ± 41	104.1 ± 4.2	113.3 ±14.8	80.7 ± 6.7	71.1 ± 8.9
K272A	C	136.2 ± 17.3	97.7 ± 1.5	88.5 ± 11.8	88.5 ± 6.5	87.6 ± 13.2
D273A	C	101.4 ± 12.8	97.7 ± 2	77.1 ± 2.7	91.5 ± 4.2	76.2 ± 15.6
L280A	***H***	***45 ± 12.2***	***90.7 ± 4.7***	***12.1 ± 7.9***	***6.1 ± 3.3***	***7.6 ± 7.1***
R282A	***C***	***80.7 ± 11.2***	***98.6 ± 0.7***	***10.1 ± 3.6***	***74.2 ± 5***	***53.5 ± 9.6***
L285A/I286A	***H***	***63.7 ± 13.5***	***98.9 ± 4.7***	***18.4 ± 5.4***	***4.2 ± 2.6***	***0.5 ± 0.5***
K291A	C	43.4 ± 15.3	90.2 ± 1.8	58.5 ± 16.2	88.5 ± 6	92.8 ± 6.8
K300A	C	49 ± 16.5	88.1 ± 0.6	77.6 ± 6.5	100.8 ± 4.9	86.4 ± 10.6
H305A	C	95.8 ± 34.7	89.6 ± 0.7	82.2 ± 1.2	53.8 ± 8.8	43.2 ± 3.9
D306A	C	98.5 ± 31.1	85.8 ± 8.3	96 ± 8.1	67.8 ± 9.6	73.2 ± 8.9
E308A	C	0 ± 0	3.0 ± 1.0	18.2 ± 8.3		
F309A	H	0 ± 0	0 ± 0	6.2 ± 2.1		
L313A	H	63.9 ± 10	97.6 ± 1.4	50.8 ± 9.3	49.5 ± 12.8	41.5 ± 8.8
R314A	C	35.7 ± 11.8	78.1 ± 5.4	56.8 ± 11.2		
K320A	C	118.6 ± 27.3	104.4 ± 3.5	96 ± 9.1	90.4 ± 3.4	75.3 ± 21
I323A	***H***	***116.4 ± 26.2***	***95.6 ± 3.5***	***20 ± 7.3***	***0.5 ± 0.3***	***0 ± 0***
L326A	H	57.3 ± 13.3	68.6 ± 8.1	84.1 ± 4.6	82.6 ± 6	73.6 ± 9.4
K327A	C	69.8 ± 12.8	93.4 ± 5.6	78.3 ± 9	95.0 ± 5.5	83.1 ± 8.7
I334A	H	18.8 ± 6.6	65 ± 8.8	84.7 ± 10		
I337A	H	12.2 ± 4.9	34.2 ± 11.5	46.5 ± 9.6		
L344A/I345A	H	0 ± 0	0 ± 0	14.7 ± 4.8		
L349A	H	54.7 ± 15.1	89.3 ± 5.8	99.1 ± 2.2	64.4 ± 12.2	76.9 ± 4.6
K352A	C	32.1 ± 8.2	87.3 ± 5.3	90.3 ± 10.7	56.5 ± 9.5	68.5 ± 9.5
H354A	C	79.9 ± 26	90.8 ± 4.3	96.9 ± 3.5	89.7 ± 4.9	92.2 ± 8.7
L355A	H	14.8 ± 4.1	53.9 ± 8.7	25.2 ± 4.9		
K356A	C	85.7 ± 37.1	93.6 ± 3.6	83.5 ± 13.3	36.8 ± 4.0	29.4 ± 5.5
D357A	C	39.4 ± 13.3	97.6 ± 2.2	40.6 ± 9.1		
I358A	H	68.2 ± 11.7	99 ± 2.3	96.3 ± 3.7	75.1 ± 8.5	66.7 ± 9.9
I361A	H	117.5 ± 28.8	106 ± 2.1	98.1 ± 3.1	21.3 ± 11	24.1 ± 7.2
K368A	C	13.6 ± 2.8	54.3 ± 10.7	32.5 ± 9.6		
L372A	H	0 ± 0	0 ± 0	17.3 ± 7.8		
L382A	H	25.6 ± 8.9	66.8 ± 6.5	72.9 ± 10.5		
K384A	C	24.2 ± 3.3	82.3 ± 9.2	64.6 ± 1.4	70.1 ± 3.3	55.1 ± 9.4
L387A	H	71.4 ± 16.4	97.4 ± 3.9	94.8 ± 10.8	43.3 ± 11.7	37.6 ± 5.9
L394A	***H***	***45.7 ± 4.9***	***93.8 ± 5.3***	***12.8 ± 6.7***	***2 ± 1***	***0 ± 0***
H398A	C	165 ± 93.7	98.7 ± 1.8	88.3 ± 14.8	90.5 ± 2.0	79.3 ± 5.6
I403A	***H***	***57.8 ± 13.7***	***94.9 ± 6.7***	***12.3 ± 8.2***	***12.4 ± 1.4***	***13.8 ± 5.4***
E404A	C	43.5 ± 19.8	97 ± 3	63.1 ± 4.3	96.3 ± 3.3	93.9 ± 2.9
I411A	H	63.7 ± 20.1	92.7 ± 6.4	38.1 ± 11.9		
L415A	***H***	***34.1 ± 10.7***	***81.3 ± 7.5***	***14.6 ± 7.8***	***0.3 ± 0.2***	***0 ± 0***
K417A	C	22.1 ± 12.4	87.3 ± 11	29.5 ± 18		
R422A	***C***	***286.2 ± 138.8***	***97 ± 5.5***	***14.6 ± 10.1***	***23.4 ± 4.1***	***19.2 ± 6.2***
H448A	C	560.5 ± 235.9	113 ± 3.7	64.9 ± 3.1	8.9 ± 5.6	9.8 ± 5.5
L449A	H	41.6 ± 16.9	82.2 ± 5	86.2 ± 8	89.3 ± 4.3	88.2 ± 7.4
K451A	C	225.4 ± 48.5	110.9 ± 1.6	84.1 ± 11.2	94.4 ± 4.9	81.3 ± 8.8
I452A	H	40.1 ± 13.5	90.8 ± 5.9	79.5 ± 10.1		
I458A	H	95.7 ± 26.7	103 ± 3.1	88.9 ± 5.2	90.9 ± 4.2	97.9 ± 5.0
K465A	C	91.6 ± 28.9	101.4 ± 6	52.7 ± 14.8	3.8 ± 1.3	11.3 ± 2.1
H467A/R468A	C	0 ± 0	0 ± 0	2.4 ± 2.4		
L469A	H	19.2 ± 3.1	81.7 ± 7.2	40.6 ± 5.9		
K481A	C	393.2 ± 200.5	112.3 ± 3.3	74.9 ± 5.2	94.9 ± 6.7	83.8 ± 11.5
K490A/R491A	C	223.7 ± 64.1	103.6 ± 1.2	91.8 ± 7.1	102.8 ± 5.1	86.8 ± 9.3

[1] Mutations that impaired GP2 function (>80% cleavage efficiency and <20% fusion activity) are bold and italicized.
[2] Table 1 abbreviations. H: Hydrophobic; C: Charged. [3] All values are displayed as a percentage of GP control ± SEM.

To determine if the charged constructs produced functional GP, we assessed the fusion activity using the cell-to-cell based fusion assay. The majority of the mutant GPs produced syncytia at levels similar to parental GP (Figure 2B), suggesting the alanine substitutions at those positions did not impede interaction with the target membrane or low-pH induced protein conformational changes. Of the constructs that were efficiently processed into GP2, only three (GP-D268A, GP-R282A, and GP-R422A) reduced fusion (<20%) compared to parental LASV GP. D268 was adjacent to the N-terminal fusion peptide and R282 was within the internal fusion-loop, suggesting these charged residues were important for GP2 to effectively anchor into the target membrane. R422 was located between HR2 and the transmembrane domain, but was not resolved in either the pre-fusion or post-fusion structures. Alanine substitution at R422 retained GP1-GP2 processing and surface expression, but the decrease in cell-to-cell fusion suggests the arginine was important for the fusion process.

2.3. Characterization of Hydrophobic Residues

Hydrophobic residues within viral class I fusion proteins are involved in protein folding and are critical for the viral fusion peptides/loops to effectively insert into the target membrane [33]. Previous studies identified hydrophobic residues within the fusion domains and C-terminus of the LASV GP2 subunit that are required for fusion [23]. We built upon this work and characterized 26 mutations throughout the GP2 subunit to identify conserved, hydrophobic residues involved in GP structure and function. Once again, we analyzed cell surface expression and cleavage of the glycoprotein constructs by purifying proteins found on the surface of transfected cells. The majority of the mutated GP proteins were cleaved, but three constructs (GP-F309A, GP-L344A/I345A, and GP-L372A) did not produce detectible GP2 (Figure 3A, Table 2). GP-L344A/I345A and GP-L372A produced the GP1GP2 protein precursor indicating the mutation prevents recognition by SKI/S1P. GP-F309A was not detected in the surface material, indicating that the mutation is deleterious to GP precursor production or trafficking (Figure 3A).

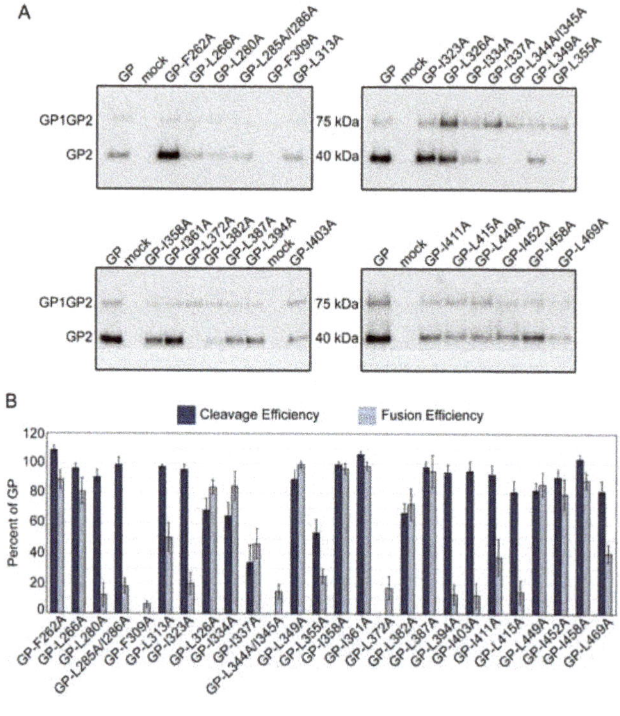

Figure 3. Functional analysis of conserved hydrophobic GP2 mutations. (**a**) Cell surface proteins were cross-linked to biotin and purified with streptavidin beads. Purified proteins were separated on SDS-PAGE and probed with anti-GP2 antibody (22.5D) representative immunoblots are shown. (**b**) LASV GP2 mutant cleavage and fusion efficiencies compared to parental GP. Error bars represent the SEM from at least three independent trials.

The cell-to-cell fusion assay results suggested many of the hydrophobic mutations reduced or eliminated syncytia formation. In total, there were six hydrophobic constructs, GP-L280A, GP-L285A/I286A, GP-I323A, GP-L394A, GP-I403A, and GP-L415A, that were efficiently cleaved (>80%) but fused <20% compared to parental LASV GP (Figure 3B). Constructs GP-L280A and GP-L285A/I286A reduced the hydrophobicity of the internal fusion loop, potentially preventing adequate insertion in the target membrane. I323 in HR1 and I403 and L415 in HR2 may have decreased efficient 6HB formation. L394 is a hydrophobic residue just outside of HR2 and may also inhibit 6HB formation.

2.4. *Transduction Efficiencies of Charged and Hydrophobic Mutants*

Our cell-to-cell fusion assay examines GP2's ability to undergo the low-pH induced conformational changes needed for fusion, but in an artificial system [34]. Lassa virus-to-cell fusion occurs in the lysosome, which contains different cellular proteins and lipids [35,36]. Therefore, to test whether the GP2 mutations affect viral entry, we pseudotyped our GP constructs onto vesicular stomatitis virus (VSV) particles lacking their native glycoprotein. VSV-LASV GP particles require LASV receptors for entry and trafficking to an endo-lysosomal compartment for efficient GP triggering. We used HAP1 and HAP1-ΔDAG haploid cell lines in our transduction assays to examine different entry mechanisms. Both cell lines have been extensively characterized for LASV entry [18,37]. HAP1 cells express the primary LASV receptor, α-dystroglycan (α-DG), and LASV entry occurs most efficiently when this receptor is present. HAP1-ΔDAG cells lack α-DG but contain secondary receptors that enable LASV entry through less efficient routes [18,31].

The LASV glycoprotein precursor must be cleaved into GP1 and GP2 to induce fusion. Therefore, we examined transduction efficiency for two sets of constructs: parental-like (constructs that produced over 80% cleaved GP2 and over 50% fusion efficiency compared to parental GP) and fusion-defective (constructs that produced over 80% cleaved GP2 but had less than 20% fusion efficiency compared to parental GP). We hypothesized that the parental-like mutants should be able to effectively transduce these cells whereas the fusion-defective mutants would have comparatively low transduction efficiencies. Because GP2 is not directly involved in receptor interactions, we expected few differences in the transduction efficiencies between HAP1 and HAP1-ΔDAG cell lines.

We examined the transduction efficiencies of 20 charged (Figure 4A, Table 2) and 10 hydrophobic parental-like constructs (Figure 4B, Table 2). The majority of the charged mutant constructs transduced cells relative to the level of GP produced in the cells. However, three constructs, GP-H305A, GP-K356A, and GP-K465A produced near wild-type levels of cleaved GP, but transduced poorly, suggesting these residues may be important in particle incorporation or fusion activity in the lysosome. Surprisingly the GP-H448A construct was unable to transduce either HAP cell line despite high cell surface production. The majority of hydrophobic constructs also transduced cells at rates similar to the levels of cleaved GP (Figure 4B). Only GP-I361A, a residue adjacent to HR-N, was cleaved and fused at parental GP levels but inefficiently transduced cells. As expected, construct transduction efficiencies did not significantly differ between cell lines, confirming that the GP2 mutations are not altering receptor interactions.

While we expected poorly-fusing mutant GPs to demonstrate equally reduced transduction, two mutant GPs, GP-D268A and GP-R282A, transduced cells efficiently (>80% and >50% respectively) (Figure 4C, Table 2). Both of these charged residues are part of the fusion peptide region; D268 is adjacent to the N-FP and R282 is within the fusion loop. The lipid and protein content of the plasma membrane and lysosomal membrane are distinct [36]. Thus, the removal of the charged residue may have altered the low-pH induced conformation of the fusion peptide, preventing proper insertion at the plasma membrane, but retaining activity in the lysosomal membrane.

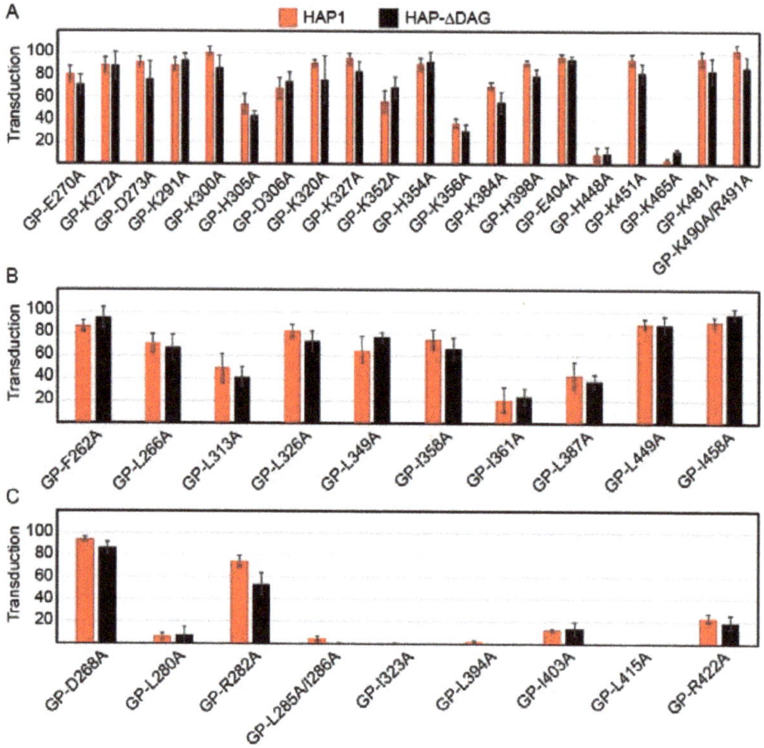

Figure 4. Transduction efficiencies of parental-like charged (**a**), parental-like hydrophobic (**b**), and fusion-defective (**c**) GP2 mutants. HAP1 and HAP1-ΔDAG1 cells were transduced with VSVΔG-LASV GP constructs encoding GFP. Transduction was quantified using flow cytometry by gating for GFP-positive cells. Transduction efficiency for each construct was normalized to parental LASV GP particle transduction for each cell line. All data are based on the average and standard error of the mean of at least three replicate experiments.

3. Discussion

In this study, we produced and characterized a library of 59 LASV GP2 mutants to identify residues involved in GP2 function. We identified 14 residues (E308, F309, I334, I337, L344/I345, L355, K368, L372, L382, K417, H467/R468, and L469) that are critical for GP folding, trafficking, or SKI/S1P recognition, evidenced by the lack of GP2 present in cell surface material. Twenty-one charged or hydrophobic residues could be changed to alanine without significantly altering protein production, localization or function, suggesting that GP2 can tolerate mutations at those locations. In total, nine constructs were efficiently cleaved (at least 80% of parental GP), yet failed to produce syncytia at levels similar to parental GP. Many of these residues, including D268, L280, R282, and L285/I286, are part of the fusion peptide domain. Both L280 and L285-I286 within I-FP impaired both cell-to-cell and virus-to-cell fusion, suggesting these hydrophobic residues may be critical for I-FP insertion, as expected (Figure 5). Surprisingly, GP-D268A and GP-R282A mutant proteins failed to induce cell-to-cell fusion, but were efficient in virus-to-cell fusion when incorporated onto VSV particles. These data suggest the charged residues are required for mediating fusion at the plasma membrane that is predominantly saturated lipids and sterols, but are less important when fusing in the lysosomal membrane, which contains low levels of cholesterol [36,38]. Similar lipid-dependent fusion occurs with other viruses; efficient insertion of the Dengue fusion peptide requires specific lipids within the late endosomes and fails to mediate low-pH fusion at the plasma membrane [39].

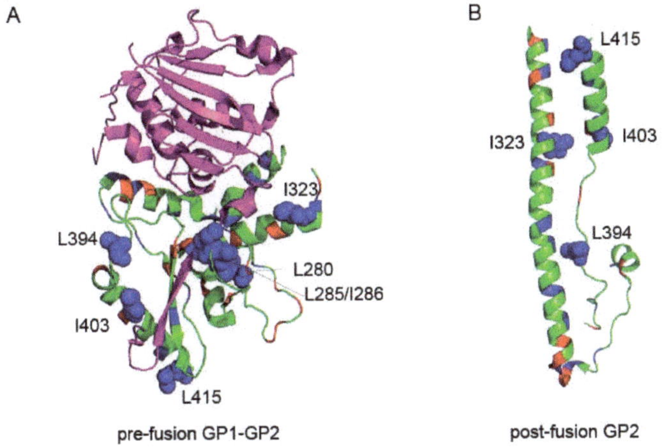

C
```
LCMV 313 EEFSDMLRLIDYNKAALSKFKQDVESALHVFKTTVNSLISDQLLMRNHLRDLMGVPYCNY
LASV 307 EEFCDMLRLFDFNKQAIQRLKAEAQMSIQLINKAVNALINDQLIMKNHLRDIMGIPYCNY
         ***:***** *:** *: * * :::: : :    ** ** ***:*:*****:**:*****

LCMV 373 SKFWYLEHAKTGETSVPKCWLVTNGSYLNETHFSDQIEQEADNMITEMLR
LASV 367 SKYWYLNHTTTGRTSLPKCWLVSNGSYLNETHFSDDIEQQADNMITEMLQ
         **:***:*  **:**:******:************:***:*********
```

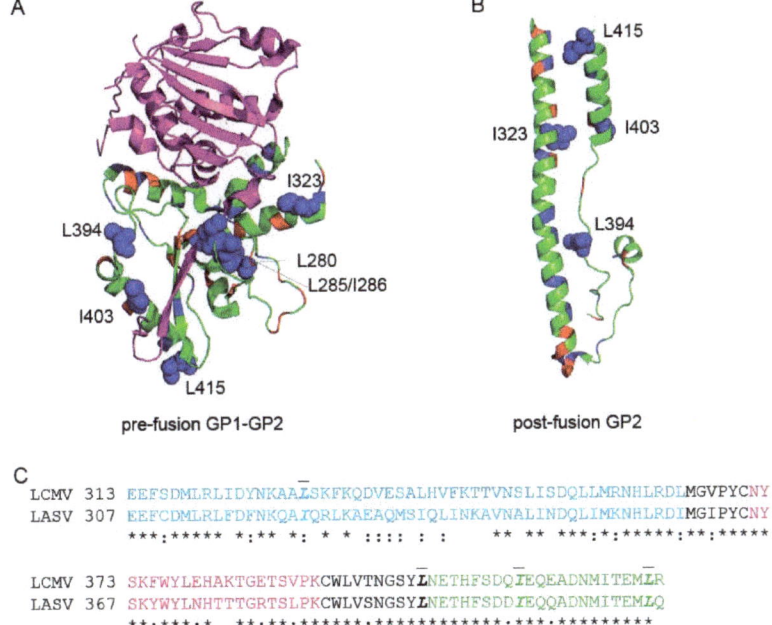

Figure 5. Mapping the fusion-defective charged and hydrophobic mutations on pre-fusion LASV GP2 and post-fusion LCMV homology model. (**a**) The LASV GP1-GP2 monomeric pre-fusion crystal structure (PDB 5vk2) [29] The GP1 subunit is shown in purple and the GP2 subunit is shown in green. The residues targeted in this study are highlighted, charged residues (red) and hydrophobic (blue). Residues found to be critical for GP2 fusion activity are shown in spheres (L280, L285/I286, I323, L394, I403, and L415) (**b**) The LCMV (an Old World arenavirus closely-related to LASV) GP2 post-fusion crystal structure (PDB 3mko) [19]. Homologous residues are highlighted as in part (a). (**c**) Amino acid alignment of LCMV GP2 region crystallized with corresponding region of LASV GP2. Identical residues are indicated with a (*), whereas conservative replacements are indicated by (:). Residues labeled in the structure are in bold-italics and contain a dash above the residues. All structures were rendered with PyMol.

While many of the residues that impacted fusion localized to the fusion peptide, five residues were part of other GP2 domains (Figure 5). I323 is part of the HR1 domain, I403 and L415 are in the HR2 domain, and L394 is the amino acid preceding HR2 (Figure 5). These residues may be critical for 6HB formation [19]. Residue R422 falls right next to the membrane but was not resolved in either crystal structure. Removal of the charged residue may impact the final 6HB structure and inhibit fusion.

Of the seven constructs that produced cleaved GP2 but failed to transduce cells (GP-L280A, GP-L285A/I286A, GP-I323A, GP-L394A, GP-I403A, GP-L415A, and GP-R422A), six were hydrophobic residues. While all of the constructs retained high cleavage efficiencies, several (GP-L280A, GP-L285A/I286A, GP-L394A, GP-I403A, and GP-L415A) produced decreased levels of GP on the surface, which may contribute to the decreased transduction.

Three of our hydrophobic constructs, GP-F262A, GP-L266A, and GP-L280A were previously characterized [23]. Klewitz et al. found GP-F262A and GP-L266A produced very little protein on the surface and had no fusion activity [23]. However, our cleavage data suggests that both GP-F262A and GP-L266A are surface-expressed near or above parental GP levels and induced both cell-to-cell and virus-to-cell fusion (Figure 3A). These phenotypic differences may be due to a difference in our transfection protocols, harvesting cells at 36 h versus 24 h, which allows more time for GP to traffic to the cell surface. We both found GP-L280A produced cleaved GP2, albeit at a decreased level, but was unable to induce fusion. Therefore, while the hydrophobic nature of the N-FP and I-FP is important, some individual residues can be made less hydrophobic while preserving functionality. Both data sets agree that the internal fusion peptide region is important for protein function.

Taken together, these data demonstrate that both conserved hydrophobic and charged residues throughout GP2 are required for optimal protein function. Specifically, the data highlighted specific residues near or within the I-FP, HR1, and HR2 domains that play critical roles in fusion.

4. Materials and Methods

Cell Lines and Transfections

Vero cells stably expressing human SLAM were maintained in Dulbecco—s modified Eagle—s medium (DMEM) with 5% (*v*/*v*) fetal bovine serum (FBS) and incubated at 37 °C and 5% CO_2 [40]. HAP1 and HAP1-ΔDAG1 cells (Horizon Discovery, Cambridge, UK) were maintained in Iscove's media supplemented with 10% (*v*/*v*) FBS and incubated at 37 °C and 5% CO_2. All transfections were performed with GeneJuice (Millipore, Burlington, MA) according to the manufacturer's instructions.

Expression Vectors and Mutagenesis

The LASV GPC protein coding sequence was codon optimized for mammalian expression and cloned into a pcDNA3.1 intron vector. A CMV promoter initiated gene expression, and we included a β-globin intron in the 5′ untranslated region (UTR) to increase protein production [31]. We added a carboxy-terminal 3xFLAG tag to the GP2 cytoplasmic tail to biochemically detect HA and charged constructs. HA insertions and point mutations were created with QuikChange mutagenesis and PfuTurbo-HS polymerase (Agilent, Santa Clara, CA). We verified the presence of each mutation with DNA sequence analysis, and a complete sequence information is available upon request.

Surface Biotinylation

Vero cells were transfected (as described above) with plasmid DNA encoding the indicated LASV GPC construct. Thirty-six hours following transfection, cells were washed with cold PBS and incubated with 0.5 mg/mL sulfosuccinimidyl-2-(biotinamido) ethyl-1,3-dithiopropionate (ThermoFisher, Waltham, MA) for 30 min on ice to tag cell surface proteins with biotin [41]. The reaction was quenched with Tris-HCl, and cells were lysed in M2 lysis buffer (50 mM Tris, pH 7.4, 150 mM NaCl, 1 mM EDTA, 1% Triton X-100) at 4°C, then centrifuged (20,000× g, 15 min, 4°C). The clarified lysate was rotated with streptavidin sepharose beads (GE Healthcare, Chicago, IL) for 60 min. Following incubation, the streptavidin sepharose beads were washed in buffer 1 (100 mM Tris, 500 mM lithium chloride, 0.1% Triton X-100) and then in buffer 2 (20 mM HEPES (pH 7.2), 2 mM EGTA, 10 mM magnesium chloride, 0.1% Triton X-100). The samples were then incubated in urea buffer (200 mM Tris, pH 6.8, 8 M urea, 5% sodium dodecyl sulfate (SDS), 0.1 mM EDTA, 0.03% bromophenol blue, 1.5% dithiothreitol) for 30 min at 55°C and analyzed using an immunoblot.

Antibodies and Immunoblots

After surface biotinylation, samples were separated by gel electrophoresis on 4-20% Nu-PAGE gels (ThermoFisher, Waltham, MA) and transferred to polyvinylidene difluoride (PVDF) membranes (GE Healthcare). HA and charged GP constructs were detected with an antibody against the Flag epitope tag (M2; Sigma, Burlington, MA) and a mouse IgG horseradish peroxidase (HRP)-conjugated secondary antibody (Jackson ImmunoResearch, West, Grove, PA). Hydrophobic constructs were detected with an antibody against LASV GP2 (22.5D), kindly provided by Dr. James Robinson (Tulane University), and a human IgG HRP-conjugated secondary antibody (Jackson). Immunoblots were visualized with SuperSignal West Dura Extended Duration Substrate (ThermoFisher, Waltham, MA) and a ChemiDoc digital imaging system (Bio-Rad, Hercules, CA). Immunoblots were quantified using ImageLab software (Bio-Rad, Hercules, CA).

Cell-to-Cell Fusion Assay

Vero cells were co-transfected with LASV GP mutants and pmaxGFP (4:1 ratio). Forty hours following transfection, media was removed and replaced with PBS (pH 4) and incubated (37 °C and 5% CO_2) for 30 min to allow glycoprotein triggering. The PBS was replaced with warm DMEM and cells were incubated for an additional 3 h to enable membrane rearrangement and syncytia formation. Four representative pictures of the fusion were taken using Zoe microscope (Bio-Rad) (20× magnification) and unfused cells were counted. Fusion efficiency was quantified using the following equation:

$$Fusion = \frac{(unfused\ cells\ in\ GFP\ transfected - unfused\ cells\ in\ mutant\ transfected)}{(unfused\ cells\ in\ GFP\ transfected - unfused\ cells\ in\ parental\ GPC\ transfected)} \times 100$$

Each mutant was assessed for fusion in at least three independent experiments.

VSV Pseudoparticle Production and Transductions

GP constructs lacking the C-terminal 3xFlag tag were used to make vesicular stomatitis virus (VSV) pseudotyped particles. Vero cells were transfected with LASV GP DNA. Thirty-six hours following transfection the cells were transduced with VSVΔG-GFP particles pseudotyped with VSV-G (MOI 1) for one hour (courtesy of Dr. Michael Whitt; KeraFAST, Boston, MA) [42]. The particle-containing media was then replaced with fresh DMEM. VSVΔG-GFP particles displaying the LASV GP were collected 8 h following the transduction. These particles were applied onto HAP1 and HAP1-ΔDAG1 cells. A larger volume of particles (4 times as much) was used to transduce HAP1-ΔDAG1 cells to overcome the decreased transduction efficiency when cells are missing the primary α-DG receptor [18]. The number of GFP positive cells was enumerated in a flow cytometer. Results are displayed as the percent of GFP positive cells present in a population of 10,000 live cell events compared to parental GP transduction.

Author Contributions: Conceptualization, M.A.B.; Methodology, M.A.B.; Validation, K.A.W., J.T.A., and M.A.B.; Formal Analysis, K.A.W., J.T.A., and M.A.B.; Investigation, K.A.W., J.T.A., M.A., and M.A.B.; Resources, M.A.B.; Data Curation, K.A.W., J.T.A., and M.A.B.; Writing-Original Draft Preparation, K.A.W. and J.T.A.; Writing—Review and Editing, K.A.W. and M.A.B.; Visualization, K.A.W. and J.T.A.; Supervision, M.A.B.; Project Administration, M.A.B.; Funding Acquisition, M.A.B.

Funding: This research was funded by The National Institutes of Health grant number [AI104800, 2015].

Acknowledgments: We thank the CVM Cytometry Core Facility for technical assistance, members of the Brindley lab for helpful comments on the manuscript, and Dr. James Robinson at Tulane University for providing antibodies against LASV GP.

Conflicts of Interest: The authors declare no conflict of interest.

References

1. Maes, P.; Alkhovsky, S.V.; Bao, Y.; Beer, M.; Birkhead, M.; Briese, T.; Buchmeier, M.J.; Calisher, C.H.; Charrel, R.N.; Choi, I.R.; et al. Taxonomy of the family Arenaviridae and the order Bunyavirales: Update 2018. *Arch. Virol.* **2018**, *163*, 2295–2310. [CrossRef] [PubMed]
2. Ogbu, O.; Ajuluchukwu, E.; Uneke, C.J. Lassa fever in West African sub-region: An overview. *J. Vector Borne Dis.* **2007**, *44*, 1–11. [PubMed]
3. Fichet-Calvet, E.; Rogers, D.J. Risk maps of Lassa fever in West Africa. *PLoS Negl. Trop. Dis.* **2009**, *3*, e388. [CrossRef] [PubMed]
4. Lassa Fever—Nigeria. Available online: http://www.who.int/csr/don/20-april-2018-lassa-fever-nigeria/en/ (accessed on 2 July 2018).
5. Olayemi, A.; Cadar, D.; Magassouba, N.; Obadare, A.; Kourouma, F.; Oyeyiola, A.; Fasogbon, S.; Igbokwe, J.; Rieger, T.; Bockholt, S.; et al. New Hosts of The Lassa Virus. *Sci. Rep.* **2016**, *6*, 25280. [CrossRef] [PubMed]

6. Monath, T.P.; Newhouse, V.F.; Kemp, G.E.; Setzer, H.W.; Cacciapuoti, A. Lassa virus isolation from Mastomys natalensis rodents during an epidemic in Sierra Leone. *Science* **1974**, *185*, 263–265. [CrossRef] [PubMed]
7. Ajayi, N.A.; Ukwaja, K.N.; Ifebunandu, N.A.; Nnabu, R.; Onwe, F.I.; Asogun, D.A. Lassa fever—Full recovery without ribavarin treatment: A case report. *Afr. Health Sci.* **2014**, *14*, 1074–1077. [CrossRef]
8. Prescott, J.B.; Marzi, A.; Safronetz, D.; Robertson, S.J.; Feldmann, H.; Best, S.M. Immunobiology of Ebola and Lassa virus infections. *Nat. Rev. Immunol.* **2017**, *17*, 195–207. [CrossRef]
9. Yun, N.E.; Walker, D.H. Pathogenesis of Lassa fever. *Viruses* **2012**, *4*, 2031–2048. [CrossRef]
10. Burri, D.J.; Pasqual, G.; Rochat, C.; Seidah, N.G.; Pasquato, A.; Kunz, S. Molecular characterization of the processing of arenavirus envelope glycoprotein precursors by subtilisin kexin isozyme-1/site-1 protease. *J. Virol.* **2012**, *86*, 4935–4946. [CrossRef]
11. Kunz, S.; Edelmann, K.H.; de la Torre, J.C.; Gorney, R.; Oldstone, M.B. Mechanisms for lymphocytic choriomeningitis virus glycoprotein cleavage, transport, and incorporation into virions. *Virology* **2003**, *314*, 168–178. [CrossRef]
12. Lenz, O.; ter Meulen, J.; Klenk, H.D.; Seidah, N.G.; Garten, W. The Lassa virus glycoprotein precursor GP-C is proteolytically processed by subtilase SKI-1/S1P. *Proc. Natl. Acad. Sci. USA* **2001**, *98*, 12701–12705. [CrossRef] [PubMed]
13. Bederka, L.H.; Bonhomme, C.J.; Ling, E.L.; Buchmeier, M.J. Arenavirus stable signal peptide is the keystone subunit for glycoprotein complex organization. *MBio* **2014**, *5*, e02063. [CrossRef] [PubMed]
14. Eichler, R.; Lenz, O.; Strecker, T.; Eickmann, M.; Klenk, H.D.; Garten, W. Identification of Lassa virus glycoprotein signal peptide as a trans-acting maturation factor. *EMBO Rep.* **2003**, *4*, 1084–1088. [CrossRef] [PubMed]
15. Eichler, R.; Lenz, O.; Strecker, T.; Garten, W. Signal peptide of Lassa virus glycoprotein GP-C exhibits an unusual length. *FEBS Lett.* **2003**, *538*, 203–206. [CrossRef]
16. Messina, E.L.; York, J.; Nunberg, J.H. Dissection of the role of the stable signal peptide of the arenavirus envelope glycoprotein in membrane fusion. *J. Virol.* **2012**, *86*, 6138–6145. [CrossRef] [PubMed]
17. Hastie, K.M.; Igonet, S.; Sullivan, B.M.; Legrand, P.; Zandonatti, M.A.; Robinson, J.E.; Garry, R.F.; Rey, F.A.; Oldstone, M.B.; Saphire, E.O. Crystal structure of the prefusion surface glycoprotein of the prototypic arenavirus LCMV. *Nat. Struct. Mol. Biol.* **2016**. [CrossRef] [PubMed]
18. Jae, L.T.; Raaben, M.; Herbert, A.S.; Kuehne, A.I.; Wirchnianski, A.S.; Soh, T.K.; Stubbs, S.H.; Janssen, H.; Damme, M.; Saftig, P.; et al. Virus entry. Lassa virus entry requires a trigger-induced receptor switch. *Science* **2014**, *344*, 1506–1510. [CrossRef] [PubMed]
19. Igonet, S.; Vaney, M.C.; Vonrhein, C.; Bricogne, G.; Stura, E.A.; Hengartner, H.; Eschli, B.; Rey, F.A. X-ray structure of the arenavirus glycoprotein GP2 in its postfusion hairpin conformation. *Proc. Natl. Acad. Sci. USA* **2011**, *108*, 19967–19972. [CrossRef] [PubMed]
20. Eschli, B.; Quirin, K.; Wepf, A.; Weber, J.; Zinkernagel, R.; Hengartner, H. Identification of an N-terminal trimeric coiled-coil core within arenavirus glycoprotein 2 permits assignment to class I viral fusion proteins. *J. Virol.* **2006**, *80*, 5897–5907. [CrossRef] [PubMed]
21. Cao, W.; Henry, M.D.; Borrow, P.; Yamada, H.; Elder, J.H.; Ravkov, E.V.; Nichol, S.T.; Compans, R.W.; Campbell, K.P.; Oldstone, M.B. Identification of alpha-dystroglycan as a receptor for lymphocytic choriomeningitis virus and Lassa fever virus. *Science* **1998**, *282*, 2079–2081. [CrossRef]
22. Glushakova, S.E.; Lukashevich, I.S.; Baratova, L.A. Prediction of arenavirus fusion peptides on the basis of computer analysis of envelope protein sequences. *FEBS Lett.* **1990**, *269*, 145–147. [CrossRef]
23. Klewitz, C.; Klenk, H.D.; ter Meulen, J. Amino acids from both N-terminal hydrophobic regions of the Lassa virus envelope glycoprotein GP-2 are critical for pH-dependent membrane fusion and infectivity. *J. Gen. Virol.* **2007**, *88*, 2320–2328. [CrossRef] [PubMed]
24. Glushakova, S.E.; Omelyanenko, V.G.; Lukashevitch, I.S.; Bogdanov, A.A., Jr.; Moshnikova, A.B.; Kozytch, A.T.; Torchilin, V.P. The fusion of artificial lipid membranes induced by the synthetic arenavirus –fusion peptide–. *Biochim. Biophys. Acta* **1992**, *1110*, 202–208. [CrossRef]
25. Li, S.; Sun, Z.; Pryce, R.; Parsy, M.L.; Fehling, S.K.; Schlie, K.; Siebert, C.A.; Garten, W.; Bowden, T.A.; Strecker, T.; et al. Acidic pH-Induced Conformations and LAMP1 Binding of the Lassa Virus Glycoprotein Spike. *PLoS Pathog.* **2016**, *12*, e1005418. [CrossRef] [PubMed]
26. Cohen-Dvashi, H.; Israeli, H.; Shani, O.; Katz, A.; Diskin, R. The role of LAMP1 binding and pH sensing by the spike complex of Lassa virus. *J. Virol.* **2016**. [CrossRef] [PubMed]

27. Hulseberg, C.E.; Feneant, L.; Szymanska, K.M.; White, J.M. Lamp1 Increases the Efficiency of Lassa Virus Infection by Promoting Fusion in Less Acidic Endosomal Compartments. *MBio* **2018**, 9. [CrossRef] [PubMed]
28. White, J.M.; Delos, S.E.; Brecher, M.; Schornberg, K. Structures and mechanisms of viral membrane fusion proteins: Multiple variations on a common theme. *Crit. Rev. Biochem. Mol. Biol.* **2008**, *43*, 189–219. [CrossRef] [PubMed]
29. Hastie, K.M.; Zandonatti, M.A.; Kleinfelter, L.M.; Heinrich, M.L.; Rowland, M.M.; Chandran, K.; Branco, L.M.; Robinson, J.E.; Garry, R.F.; Saphire, E.O. Structural basis for antibody-mediated neutralization of Lassa virus. *Science* **2017**, *356*, 923–928. [CrossRef]
30. York, J.; Nunberg, J.H. A novel zinc-binding domain is essential for formation of the functional Junin virus envelope glycoprotein complex. *J. Virol.* **2007**, *81*, 13385–13391. [CrossRef]
31. Acciani, M.; Alston, J.T.; Zhao, G.; Reynolds, H.; Ali, A.M.; Xu, B.; Brindley, M.A. Mutational Analysis of Lassa Virus Glycoprotein Highlights Regions Required for Alpha-Dystroglycan Utilization. *J. Virol.* **2017**, *91*. [CrossRef]
32. Aftabuddin, M.; Kundu, S. Hydrophobic, hydrophilic, and charged amino acid networks within protein. *Biophys. J.* **2007**, *93*, 225–231. [CrossRef] [PubMed]
33. Apellaniz, B.; Huarte, N.; Largo, E.; Nieva, J.L. The three lives of viral fusion peptides. *Chem. Phys. Lipids* **2014**, *181*, 40–55. [CrossRef] [PubMed]
34. Mindell, J.A. Lysosomal acidification mechanisms. *Annu. Rev. Physiol.* **2012**, *74*, 69–86. [CrossRef] [PubMed]
35. Van Meer, G. Transport and sorting of membrane lipids. *Curr. Opin. Cell Biol.* **1993**, *5*, 661–673. [CrossRef]
36. Holthuis, J.C.; Menon, A.K. Lipid landscapes and pipelines in membrane homeostasis. *Nature* **2014**, *510*, 48–57. [CrossRef] [PubMed]
37. Jae, L.T.; Raaben, M.; Riemersma, M.; van Beusekom, E.; Blomen, V.A.; Velds, A.; Kerkhoven, R.M.; Carette, J.E.; Topaloglu, H.; Meinecke, P.; et al. Deciphering the glycosylome of dystroglycanopathies using haploid screens for lassa virus entry. *Science* **2013**, *340*, 479–483. [CrossRef] [PubMed]
38. Schoer, J.K.; Gallegos, A.M.; McIntosh, A.L.; Starodub, O.; Kier, A.B.; Billheimer, J.T.; Schroeder, F. Lysosomal membrane cholesterol dynamics. *Biochemistry* **2000**, *39*, 7662–7677. [CrossRef]
39. Zaitseva, E.; Yang, S.T.; Melikov, K.; Pourmal, S.; Chernomordik, L.V. Dengue virus ensures its fusion in late endosomes using compartment-specific lipids. *PLoS Pathog.* **2010**, *6*, e1001131. [CrossRef]
40. Ono, N.; Tatsuo, H.; Hidaka, Y.; Aoki, T.; Minagawa, H.; Yanagi, Y. Measles viruses on throat swabs from measles patients use signaling lymphocytic activation molecule (CDw150) but not CD46 as a cellular receptor. *J. Virol.* **2001**, *75*, 4399–4401. [CrossRef]
41. Brindley, M.A.; Plattet, P.; Plemper, R.K. Efficient replication of a paramyxovirus independent of full zippering of the fusion protein six-helix bundle domain. *Proc. Natl. Acad. Sci. USA* **2014**, *111*, E3795–E3804. [CrossRef]
42. Whitt, M.A. Generation of VSV pseudotypes using recombinant DeltaG-VSV for studies on virus entry, identification of entry inhibitors, and immune responses to vaccines. *J. Virol. Methods* **2010**, *169*, 365–374. [CrossRef] [PubMed]

pathogens

MDPI

Communication

Host-Driven Phosphorylation Appears to Regulate the Budding Activity of the Lassa Virus Matrix Protein

Christopher M. Ziegler [1], Philip Eisenhauer [1], Inessa Manuelyan [1,2], Marion E. Weir [3,†], Emily A. Bruce [1], Bryan A. Ballif [3] and Jason Botten [1,4,*]

1 Department of Medicine, Division of Immunobiology, University of Vermont, Burlington, VT 05405, USA; cziegler@uvm.edu (C.M.Z.); philip.eisenhauer@med.uvm.edu (P.E.); Inessa.Manuelyan@uvm.edu (I.M.); Emily.Bruce@med.uvm.edu (E.A.B.)

2 Cellular, Molecular and Biomedical Sciences Graduate Program, University of Vermont, Burlington, VT 05405, USA

3 Department of Biology, University of Vermont, Burlington, VT 05405, USA; marion.weir@cellsignal.com (M.E.W.); bballif@uvm.edu (B.A.B.)

4 Department of Microbiology and Molecular Genetics, University of Vermont, Burlington, VT 05405, USA

* Correspondence: jbotten@uvm.edu; Tel.: +1-802-656-9795

† Current address: Cell Signaling Technology, 32 Tozer Rd, Beverly, MA 01915, USA

Received: 20 November 2018; Accepted: 6 December 2018; Published: 9 December 2018

Abstract: Lassa mammarenavirus (LASV) is an enveloped RNA virus that can cause Lassa fever, an acute hemorrhagic fever syndrome associated with significant morbidity and high rates of fatality in endemic regions of western Africa. The arenavirus matrix protein Z has several functions during the virus life cycle, including coordinating viral assembly, driving the release of new virus particles, regulating viral polymerase activity, and antagonizing the host antiviral response. There is limited knowledge regarding how the various functions of Z are regulated. To investigate possible means of regulation, mass spectrometry was used to identify potential sites of phosphorylation in the LASV Z protein. This analysis revealed that two serines (S18, S98) and one tyrosine (Y97) are phosphorylated in the flexible N- and C-terminal regions of the protein. Notably, two of these sites, Y97 and S98, are located in (Y97) or directly adjacent to (S98) the PPXY late domain, an important motif for virus release. Studies with non-phosphorylatable and phosphomimetic Z proteins revealed that these sites are important regulators of the release of LASV particles and that host-driven, reversible phosphorylation may play an important role in the regulation of LASV Z protein function.

Keywords: Lassa virus; Z protein; late domain; PPXY; budding; release; matrix protein; phosphorylation; arenavirus; mass spectrometry

1. Introduction

The *Mammarenavirus* genus is comprised primarily of rodent-borne viruses, several of which are capable of causing severe hemorrhagic fever syndromes in humans [1]. Lassa virus (LASV), the causative agent of Lassa fever, is carried primarily by the multimammate rat, *Mastomys natalensis*, but other carrier rodents have been identified recently [2–4]. LASV infects up to an estimated 300,000 people each year in western Africa following exposure to rodent excreta or through hunting and consumption of infected rats [2,5–8]. Lassa virus can also spread person-to-person through direct contact with infected bodily fluids, and this pattern of transmission has occurred repeatedly in hospital workers caring for Lassa fever patients since its discovery in 1969 [9–11]. Overall, the case fatality rate is estimated at 1–2%, but significantly higher rates of fatality occur in hospitalized patients [5]. Since 2008, outbreaks in Sierra Leone have resulted in an overall case fatality rate of 69% in hospitalized patients [12]. LASV infection results in fetal loss in most cases [13]. Further, pregnancy greatly increases the risk of fatality from Lassa fever for the mother [13]. Of Lassa fever survivors who were hospitalized, approximately one-third developed hearing loss, and in two-thirds of those patients, the hearing deficit was permanent [14]. Intravenous ribavirin treatment has been shown to reduce mortality from Lassa fever, particularly if administered during the first six days of fever onset, but there is a clear need for more effective therapies [5]. No United States Food and Drug Administration (FDA)-approved vaccines exist for the prevention of LASV infection.

Arenaviruses have a simple, negative-strand RNA genome that encodes a total of four proteins on two segments. The small (S) segment encodes both the nucleoprotein (NP), which encapsidates the viral genome and is required for its replication, and the envelope glycoprotein (GP), which interacts with cell surface receptors to mediate cell entry and membrane fusion [15–20]. The large (L) genome segment encodes the viral RNA-dependent RNA polymerase (L), which replicates and transcribes the genome, and the viral matrix protein (Z) [19–22]. The Z protein is a structural component of the virion, forming a matrix layer on the inner leaflet of the viral envelope, and carries out an array of important functions during viral propagation [23,24]. The Z protein of pathogenic arenaviruses antagonizes interferon production by binding to retinoic acid-inducible gene I (RIG-I) and melanoma differentiation-associated protein 5 (MDA5) to disrupt interactions between RIG-I-like receptors and mitochondrial antiviral signaling (MAVS) [25]. Z can inhibit the translation of capped cellular mRNAs and also regulate the activity of the viral polymerase [26–28]. Z is also an important coordinator of virus particle assembly by interacting with each of the other three viral proteins [29,30].

In addition to these functions, the Z protein is both necessary and sufficient for driving the efficient release of nascent virus particles [23,31,32]. However, minimal levels of virus can be recovered without Z [33]. Two major motifs in the Z protein mediate the efficient release of virus particles. First, a myristoylation modification of the second residue in Z, a glycine, mediates Z's interaction with cellular membranes, a requirement for efficient release [34,35]. Second, all arenavirus Z proteins, with the exception of the Tacaribe virus Z protein, contain one or two proline-rich, late domains near the C-terminus [23,32]. These viral late domains are presumably responsible for recruiting the cellular endosomal sorting complex required for transport (ESCRT) pathway to mediate membrane scission, which is the final step in the virus budding process [36]. New World arenavirus Z proteins contain a P(S/T)AP-type late domain, which can bind the ESCRT-I protein Tsg101, while the Old World Z proteins of the lymphocytic choriomeningitis virus (LCMV) and Dandenong virus contain only a PPXY late domain, which can bind Nedd4-family E3 ubiquitin ligases [23,24,32,37]. Additionally, the Z proteins of several Old World arenaviruses, including Lassa, Mobala, Mopeia, and Ippy viruses, encode both the PPXY and the P(S/T)AP late domains [23,24,32]. In the case of LASV, decreased virus-like particle (VLP) release occurs following mutation of either of LASV Z's PTAP and PPXY late domains, disruption of Z's recruitment of Nedd4-family proteins, and/or loss of specific ESCRT components [23,24,32,37–39]. The release of VLPs for the related Old World arenavirus LCMV is similarly impacted by PPXY late domain or ESCRT component disruption [32]. However, recent work from our lab demonstrated that in a whole virus system, the sole late domain in the LCMV Z protein and the ESCRT pathway it recruits were specifically required for the production of defective interfering particles but not of infectious virus [40]. This illustrates the complexity and diversity in arenavirus release and highlights the need for a greater understanding of the factors involved in this process.

Protein phosphorylation is a reversible post-translational modification that can regulate the activity of enzymes, mediate protein–protein interactions, alter the subcellular localization, conformation, and/or oligomeric state of proteins, as well as regulate the addition or removal of other types of post-translation modifications [41]. This important type of modification is not limited to cellular proteins; a growing body of literature has demonstrated that phosphorylation of viral proteins has important consequences for different viral processes [42–45]. Phosphorylation sites of functional significance have been identified on the matrix proteins in an array of RNA viruses, including the Z protein of the Old World arenavirus LCMV [40,46–51]. Accordingly, we hypothesized that the functionality of the LASV Z protein may be regulated by phosphorylation. To address this hypothesis, mass spectrometry was used to identify phosphorylated residues in LASV Z. This approach revealed three sites of phosphorylation, including two phosphorylated serines and one tyrosine. A VLP release assay demonstrated that serine phosphorylation may negatively impact virus release. These findings are an important first step toward understanding how various functions of the LASV Z protein can be regulated by post-translational modifications.

2. Results and Discussion

To identify sites of phosphorylation, LASV Z protein was affinity purified from VLPs produced from plasmid-transfected cells and subjected to protein gel electrophoresis (Figure 1A). The gel band corresponding to LASV Z was excised and proteolytically digested. The resulting peptides were analyzed by liquid chromatography–tandem mass spectrometry. Three phosphorylated residues in the LASV Z protein were identified: two serine residues (S18 and S98) and one tyrosine residue (Y97) (Figure 1B, Figures S1 and S2). Representative mass spectra and the accompanying fragment ion tables for peptides harboring phosphorylated Y97 (Figure S1A), phosphorylated S98 (Figure S1C), as well as corresponding unphosphorylated peptides are shown (Figure S1B). Representative mass spectra and corresponding fragment ion tables of the peptides harboring phosphorylated S18 (Figure S2A) and unphosphorylated S18 (Figure S2B) are shown.

Each phosphorylation site was mapped onto the NMR structure of LASV Z (Figure 1B) [52]. The arenavirus Z protein is comprised of a central zinc-binding, really interesting new gene (RING) domain flanked by N- and C-terminal domains that appear to be flexible and relatively unstructured [52–57]. All three phosphorylation sites identified are located in these flexible N-terminal (S18) or C-terminal (Y97 and S98) domains of the Z protein (Figure 1B,C) [52]. The N-terminal domain of Z is known to mediate several important functions. It contains a myristoylation site at the second glycine residue which is required for virus budding as well as Z's interaction with the plasma membrane and with the envelope glycoprotein [30,34,35]. Other conserved residues in the N-terminal domain contribute to the production of infectious virus-like particles [58]. Additionally, the N-terminal domain of pathogenic arenaviruses, including LASV, but not of non-pathogenic arenaviruses, can directly bind to and inhibit the function of retinoic acid-inducible gene 1-like receptors (RLRs), which results in decreased macrophage activation [25,59]. The Clustal Omega multiple sequence alignment tool was used to align select mammarenavirus Z proteins (Figure 1C) [60]. This revealed that the S18 phosphorylation site is conserved across LASV strains representing lineages III–VI, as well as in Mobala virus and the New World Oliveros virus (Figure 1C) [61–63]. Notably, a histidine residue is found at this position in multiple lineage II LASV isolates that have recently been sequenced [64]. Interestingly, aspartic acid and glutamic acid, which are negatively charged at a physiological pH similar to phosphate, are substituted for S18 in a number of other New and Old World arenavirus Z proteins, suggesting that a negative charge at this position may be important for Z functionality (Figure 1C).

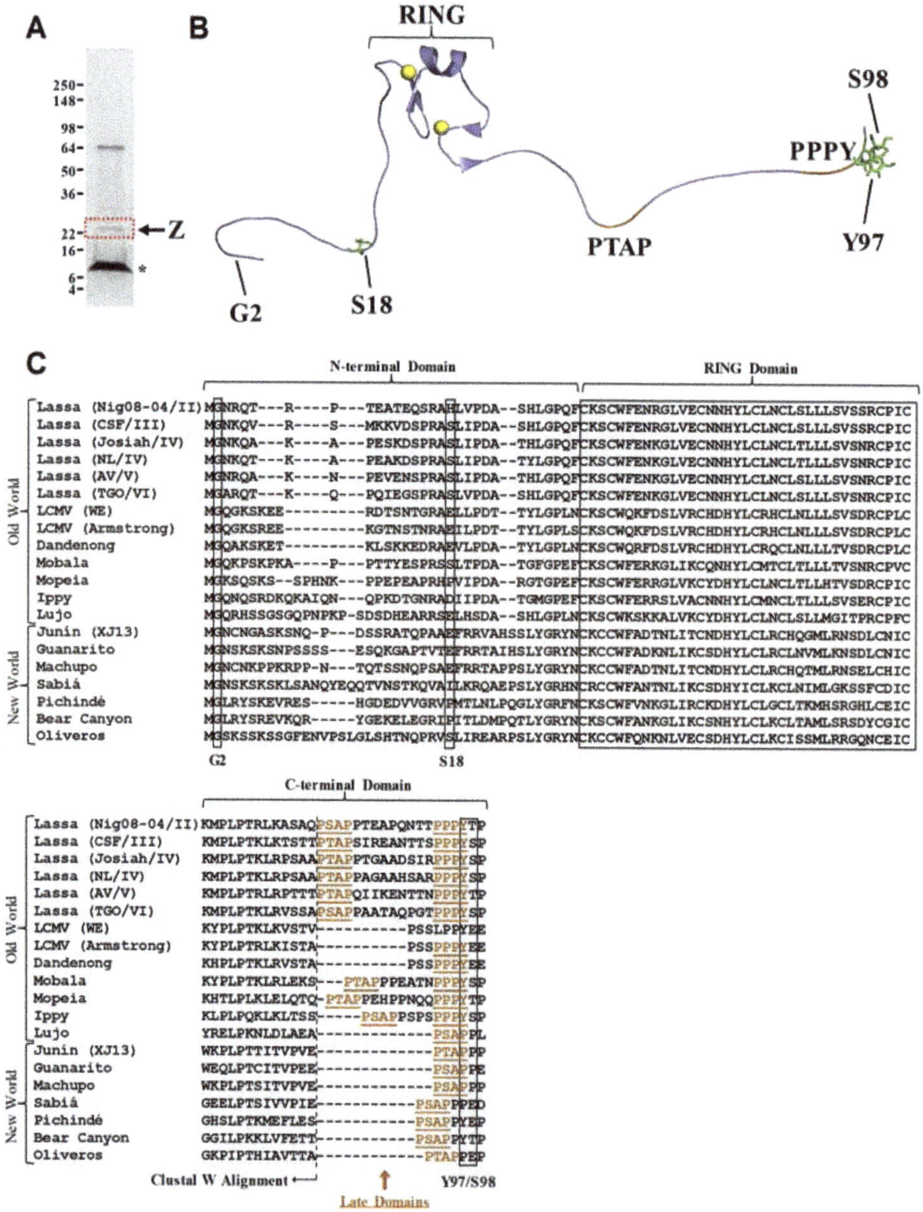

Figure 1. Identification of phosphorylation sites in the Lassa mammarenavirus (LASV) Z matrix protein. (**A**) Coomassie-stained polyacrylamide gel of affinity-purified LASV Z. Streptavidin-coated magnetic beads were used to affinity purify Z from virus-like particles (VLPs) released from cells co-transfected with plasmids encoding a biotin ligase and LASV Z C-terminally tagged with a biotin acceptor peptide (BAP). The band corresponding to the LASV Z protein (indicated by the red box) was excised from the gel and subjected to proteolytic digestion with trypsin or a combination of trypsin and chymotrypsin.

The resultant peptides were extracted and subjected to liquid chromatography–tandem mass spectrometry analysis. The asterisk denotes the band of monomeric streptavidin that is eluted from streptavidin beads following boiling. (**B**) The protein nuclear magnetic resonance structure of the Josiah strain of the LASV Z matrix (PDB 2M1S) is shown. The side chains of the phosphorylated residues (S18, Y97, and S98) are highlighted in green on the protein structure. The two late domains found in LASV Z, PTAP and PPPY, are colored orange. Zinc ions, which are coordinated by the central really interesting new gene (RING) domain of Z, are shown as yellow spheres in the protein structure. The myristoylated glycine residue (at position 2) is also indicated. (**C**) Protein sequence alignment of select mammarenavirus Z proteins. The Clustal Omega multiple sequence alignment tool was used to align the sequences of selected mammarenavirus Z proteins. The portion of the C-terminal region of each Z protein (the amino acids to the right of the dashed vertical line) containing the late domains (designated as orange, underlined amino acids) was aligned with LASV Z strain Josiah, starting with the most C-terminal amino acid. The following accession numbers were used: GU481069.1 (Lassa mammarenavirus, strain Nig08-04), AAO59514.1 (Lassa mammarenavirus, strain CSF), NP_694871.1 (Lassa mammarenavirus, strain Josiah), AAO59510.1 (Lassa mammarenavirus, strain NL), AAO59508.1 (Lassa mammarenavirus, strain AV), MF990887.1 (Lassa mammarenavirus, strain TGO) AAD03395.1 (Lymphocytic choriomeningitis mammarenavirus, strain WE), ABC96003.1 (Lymphocytic choriomeningitis mammarenavirus, strain Armstrong 53b), ABY20731.1 (Dandenong virus), ABC71138.1 (Mobala mammarenavirus), ABC71136.1 (Mopeia mammarenavirus, strain Mozambique), ABC71142.1 (Ippy mammarenavirus), YP_002929492.1 (Lujo mammarenavirus), NP_899216.1 (Junín mammarenavirus, strain XJ13), NP_899220.1 (Guanarito mammarenavirus), NP_899214.1 (Machupo mammarenavirus), ABY59837.1 (Brazilian mammarenavirus), YP_138535.1 (Pichindé mammarenavirus), YP_001649224.1 (Bear Canyon mammarenavirus), YP_001649215.1 (Oliveros mammarenavirus). For each LASV isolate, the corresponding lineage is listed after the strain.

The Y97 and S98 phosphorylation sites lie within the C-terminal tail of the LASV Z protein, a region which contains two proline-rich late domains, PTAP and PPPY (Figure 1B,C). The C-terminal amino acids containing the late domains of selected mammarenavirus Z proteins were aligned (Figure 1C). This analysis showed that Y97 is conserved across the majority of Old World mammarenaviruses (except for Lujo virus) and aligns with Pichindé and Bear Canyon New World mammarenaviruses (Figure 1C). Conservation of a serine or threonine at residues that align with LASV Z S98 is fairly common among Old World mammarenaviruses (Figure 1C). Notably, LCMV possesses a glutamic acid at this position which could substitute for the negative charge of a phosphorylated serine (Figure 1C). However, LASV Z S98 is directly followed by a proline residue. Interestingly, phosphorylated serine or threonine residues directly preceding a proline (pS/T–P) constitute a type of motif that can be recognized by class IV WW domains, including the peptidylprolyl cis/trans isomerase, NIMA-interacting 1 protein (Pin1) [65,66]. Pin1 can mediate conformational changes in substrate proteins that result in altered protein stability or phosphorylation state [67]. Because Pin1 has been implicated in different viral infections and has been shown to bind pS/T–P motifs within viral proteins from hepatitis B virus [68], human T-cell leukemia virus type 1 [69,70], human immunodeficiency virus 1 [71–73], Epstein–Barr virus [74], and Kaposi's sarcoma-associated herpesvirus [75], it may represent an interesting host target for further study in the context of the arenavirus Z protein.

The Y97 phosphorylation site lies within the PPXY late domain, which is conserved across the majority of Old World arenavirus Z proteins (Figure 1C). Our lab recently showed that the homologous tyrosine residue (Y88) in LCMV Z is also phosphorylated [40]. Treating cells with H_2O_2 to block tyrosine phosphatases and permit the accumulation of tyrosines phosphorylated by endogenous kinases demonstrated that both LCMV and LASV Z are phosphorylated on a tyrosine residue (Figure 2A) [76]. This strategy further showed that the phosphotyrosine levels of LASV Z were significantly reduced in the Y97F mutant of LASV Z, indicating that this late domain-embedded tyrosine is likely the major tyrosine phosphorylation site (Figure 2B), similar to what we observed for the PPXY-embedded Y88 in the case of LCMV [40].

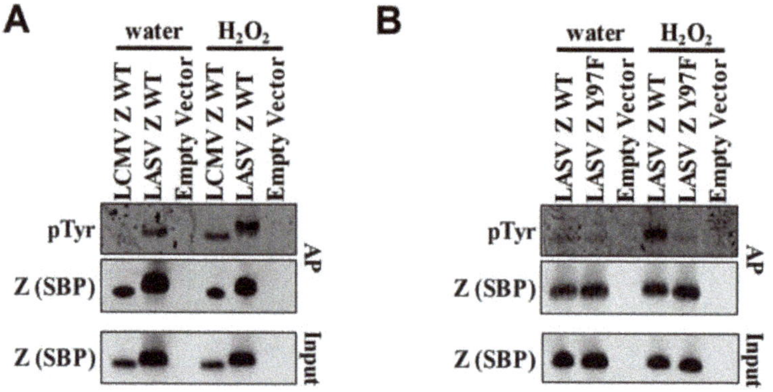

Figure 2. Confirmation of Y97 phosphorylation site in LASV Z. (**A**,**B**) HEK293T cells were transfected with plasmids encoding the indicated streptavidin-binding peptide (SBP)-tagged lymphocytic choriomeningitis virus (LCMV) Z or LASV Z, and two days later streptavidin-coated magnetic beads were used to affinity purify (AP) intracellular Z from cells that had been treated with water or hydrogen peroxide (H_2O_2). Levels of phosphotyrosine and Z-SBP in affinity-purified samples (and unpurified cellular input for Z-SBP) were determined by western blotting with anti-phosphotyrosine or anti-SBP antibodies, respectively. Levels of phosphotyrosine are shown for wild-type (WT) LCMV Z and LASV Z (**A**) as well as for WT and phosphosite-mutant (Y97F) LASV Z proteins (**B**). Western blots are representative of five (**A**) or four (**B**) independent experiments.

A prominent function of the arenavirus Z protein is to drive the release of virus particles. We next sought to determine whether any of the three phosphorylation sites might contribute to the ability of Z to drive virus budding using a VLP release assay (Figure 3A–C). For the phosphoserine residues at S18 or S98, LASV Z protein mutants encoding either an alanine or an aspartic acid substitution at these positions were made in order to prevent or to possibly mimic phosphorylation at the site in question, respectively. Phosphomimetic substitution did not result in a significant change in VLP release for either S18 or S98 (Figure 3A,C). However, substitution with alanine to either phosphoserine site resulted in levels of VLP release that were 1.5- or 2-fold greater than in the WT, suggesting that serine phosphorylation may negatively regulate the release of virus particles (Figure 3A). It is important to note that, in many cases, aspartic acid and glutamic acid do not functionally mimic phosphorylation, particularly when a phosphorylated residue is recognized by an adaptor protein [77]. Our results here could be explained if cellular kinases impinged on viral budding by promoting a phosphoserine-dependent protein–protein interaction, one which cannot be mimicked by the shape or charge afforded by aspartic acid.

For the Y97 phosphosite, phenylalanine and glutamic acid mutants were generated, again to prevent or mimic phosphorylation, respectively. Release of VLPs from cells transfected with LASV Z containing either the non-phosphorylatable (F) or phosphomimetic (E) amino acid at residue 97 was decreased by roughly 50% compared to wild-type Z-containing cells (Figure 3B,C). Given that Y97 lies within the PPXY late domain, which has been previously shown to be required for efficient release of LCMV and LASV VLPs, the results were not surprising [23,32,40] and may indicate a cellular mechanism at play to regulate viral budding. Mutation of the canonical PPXY motif in LASV results in a loss of binding to Nedd4-family E3 ubiquitin ligases, which have been implicated in the release of several other viruses that have a PPXY domain in their matrix protein [24,36]. However, in earlier work with LCMV, despite a reduction in VLP release, disruption of the PPXY late domain did not block the efficient release of infectious virus particles but rather that of defective interfering (DI) particles [40]. Furthermore, greater levels of DI particles were released with recombinant LCMV containing a glutamic acid substitution at its Y88 phosphorylation site relative to the Y88F-mutant virus, suggesting that phosphorylation may positively regulate the release of DI particles [40]. These data raise the intriguing question of whether a similar phenomenon (e.g., whereby phosphorylation of the PPXY late domain regulates the release of a specific class of viral particles) may be occurring with the LASV Z protein. There is currently little data confirming the presence of LASV DI particles. However, it is thought that most animal viruses produce some level of DI particles, and some arenaviruses in particular are known to produce significant levels of DI particles [78,79]. More specifically, a high multiplicity of infection with LASV virus yields lower infectious titers and higher ratios of viral genomic RNA to particles compared with low-multiplicity infections [80]. These findings are consistent with a virus that produces appreciable levels of DI particles [81,82].

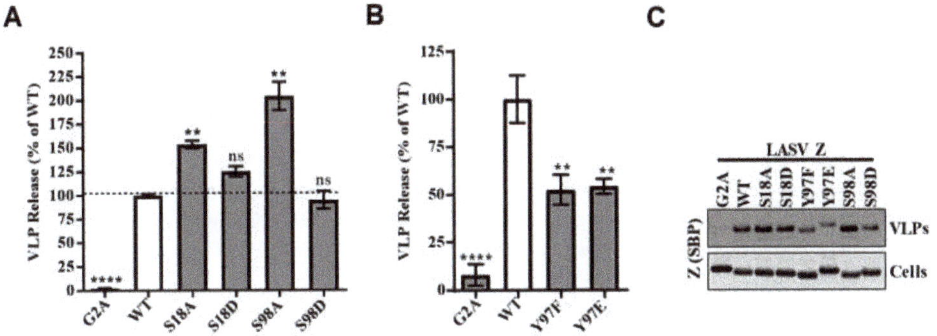

Figure 3. VLP release assay of WT and phosphomutant LASV Z proteins. (**A–C**) HEK293T cells were transfected with plasmids encoding the WT LASV Z protein or the LASV Z containing mutations that prevent (S to A; Y to F) or mimic (S to D; Y to E) phosphorylation at the serine phosphorylation sites (**A**) or the tyrosine phosphorylation site (**B**). The glycine-to-alanine mutant (G2A) served as a negative control as it prevents myristoylation of Z, resulting in drastic inhibition of Z's budding activity. Quantitative, fluorescent western blotting was used to quantify the amount of intracellular and VLP-derived Z protein. A representative western blot of intracellular or VLP-derived SBP-tagged Z protein is shown in (**C**). The VLP release activity was determined by dividing the quantity of Z in VLPs by the quantity of intracellular Z, then normalized to the amount of wild-type Z. The values represent the mean ± standard error of the mean from three (**A**) or four (**B**) independent experiments. Mean values were compared using a one-way ANOVA with the Holm–Sidak's test for multiple comparisons. (**A**,**B**), n.s. (not significant), ** $p < 0.01$, **** $p < 0.0001$.

The discovery of these phosphorylation sites opens up several new avenues for inquiry, including identifying the host kinases involved as well as any phosphosite-binding proteins that may regulate Z protein function. Kinase prediction algorithms could be used to narrow the possible candidate kinases, but empirical screens will be required to determine the kinase(s) that contribute most substantially to Z phosphorylation. Kinase identification for the LASV Z Y97 phosphosite may be aided by evidence in the literature implicating Src family or Abl tyrosine kinases in the phosphorylation of PPXY domains in other proteins—specifically, the Ebola virus matrix protein and the cellular proteins dystroglycan and IFITM3 [46,83,84]. It has also been shown for dystroglycan and IFITM3 that phosphorylation of PPXY motifs can regulate the binding of proteins that contain SH2 domains as well as of the Nedd4-family ubiquitin ligases that bind PPXY domains through their WW domain [83–85]. It is plausible that Old World mammarenavirus Z proteins are regulated in a similar fashion. It will also be important to identify phosphoserine-specific binding proteins (e.g., perhaps Pin1) or proteins containing other phosphoserine-binding domains in order to understand the mechanism by which serine phosphorylation regulates Z protein function [66]. Furthermore, it will be important to determine whether the S18 phosphorylation site or other residues in the N-terminal domain, that are more highly conserved among pathogenic arenaviruses, are involved in the inhibition of RLR signaling and macrophage activation [25,59]. Finally, the clustering of two phosphorylation sites at the C-terminus of the LASV Z protein, spanning two distinct WW domain-binding motifs, contributes to the idea that this region of Z and its corresponding functions may be intricately regulated by a network of distinct host protein partners.

3. Materials and Methods

3.1. Cells and Plasmids

Human embryonic kidney cells (HEK-293T/17, CRL-11268), purchased from American Type Culture Collection (Manassas, VA, USA), were cultured in Dulbecco's Modified Eagle Medium (DMEM) (11965-092) supplemented with 10% fetal bovine serum (FBS) (16140-071) and 1% of penicillin/streptomycin (15140-122), MEM Non-Essential Amino Acids Solution (11140-050), HEPES Buffer Solution (15630-130), and GlutaMAX (35050-061) purchased from Thermo Fisher Scientific (Carlsbad, CA, USA).

Plasmid LASV Z HA-BAP expresses the LASV Z gene from strain Josiah (GenBank #HQ688675.1) with a C-terminal hemagglutinin (HA) affinity tag followed by a tobacco etch virus cleavage site and a biotinylation acceptor peptide in a modified pCAGGS expression vector, as previously described [86, 87]. Plasmid LASV Z WT SBP is comprised of the LASV Z gene C-terminally fused to a six-amino acid linker (AAGGGG) followed by the streptavidin-binding peptide (SBP) affinity tag in a modified pCAGGS vector, as previously described [88]. Genes encoding point mutants of LASV Z (S18A, S18D, Y97F, Y97E, S98A, and S98D) were synthesized and subcloned into the LASV Z WT SBP vector by BioBasic, Inc. (Markham, ON, Canada). Plasmids expressing the Armstrong 53b strain of LCMV Z (GenBank #AY847351.1) with a C-terminal SBP tag have been described previously [40], as has the plasmid encoding the biotin ligase (BirA) [87].

3.2. Identification of Phosphorylation Sites by Mass Spectrometry

To identify potential phosphorylation sites in LASV Z, 1×10^6 HEK293T cells/well were seeded into two six-well plates. After 24 h, each well was transfected with 100 µL DMEM containing 1 µg of LASV Z HA-BAP, 1 µg of plasmid BirA, and 10 µg of polyethyleneinimine (23966, Polysciences, Inc., Warrington, PA, USA). After 48 h, the VLP-containing culture media was collected and clarified by centrifugation, then a solution of 1x Triton lysis buffer (0.5% NP40, 1% Triton X-100 (BP151-100, Fisher Scientific), 140 mM NaCl, 25 mM Tris HCl) with protease (04693159001, Roche, Indianapolis, IN, USA) and phosphatase inhibitor cocktails (4906837001, Roche) was added to lyse the VLPs. Biotin-modified LASV Z protein was affinity purified by incubating the VLP lysate with Dynabeads MyOne Streptavidin T1 beads (65602, Thermo Fisher Scientific) for 2 h at 4 °C while rotating. Following incubation, the beads were washed with 1x Triton lysis buffer and then were eluted in 4x Laemmli sample buffer (250 mM Tris-HCl, 40% glycerol, 8% sodium dodecyl sulfate, and 0.04% bromophenol blue) diluted to 1x in Triton lysis buffer with a final concentration of 5% 2-mercaptoethanol by heating at 100 °C for 10 min. The protein eluate was subjected to electrophoresis on a 4–20% Tris-glycine polyacrylamide gel (EC60285BOX, Invitrogen, Carlsbad, CA, USA). This gel was then stained overnight with Coomassie (40% methanol, 20% acetic acid, and 0.1% Brilliant Blue R (B7920, Sigma-Aldrich, St. Louis, MI, USA) followed by de-staining with a solution of 30% methanol and 10% acetic acid and was imaged on a Canon Canoscan 8800F scanner. The region of the gel lane containing the Z protein was excised and either directly reduced and alkylated with iodoacetamide or not, prior to being subjected to in-gel digestion with a solution of sequencing-grade modified trypsin (V5111, Promega, Madison, WI, USA) or a mixture of trypsin and sequencing-grade chymotrypsin (V1061, Promega), as described previously [40,51]. The resultant peptides were extracted from the gel slice using 2.5% formic acid in 50% acetonitrile and centrifugation. This supernatant was collected, and the gel slice was further dehydrated by incubating with 100% acetonitrile, centrifuging, and collecting the supernatant twice. The solvent was evaporated using a vacuum centrifuge at 37 °C, and the peptides were resuspended in 2.5% acetonitrile and 2.5% formic acid. Liquid chromatography was conducted using a microcapillary column packed with 12 cm Magic C18, 200 Å, 5 μm material (PM5/66100/00, Michrom Bioresources, Auburn, CA, USA) using a MicroAS autosampler (Thermo Scientific, Pittsburgh, PA, USA). The peptides were eluted with a gradient of 5–35% acetonitrile (0.15% formic acid) using a Surveyor Pump Plus HPLC (Thermo Scientific) over 40 min after a 15 min isocratic loading at 2.5% acetonitrile and 0.15% formic acid. Data were acquired in both a stand-alone linear ion trap mass spectrometer (LTQ-XL) and a linear ion trap–orbitrap (LTQ–Orbitrap) hybrid mass spectrometer (both instruments from Thermo Scientific). Ten MS/MS scans in the LTQ followed each linear ion trap or orbitrap survey scan over the entire run. A concatenated database of the LASV Z protein sequence including affinity tags in forward and reverse orientation was queried with SEQUEST software with no enzyme requirement and a 20 PPM precursor mass tolerance (or 2 Da for data collected in the stand-alone LTQ). The following differential modifications were allowed: +79.96633 Da for phosphorylation of serine, threonine, and tyrosine; +15.99492 Da for methionine oxidation; and either 71.0371 Da for cysteine acrylamidation or +57.02146 for cysteine carbamidomethylation.

3.3. *Detection of Phosphoproteins by Western Blotting*

In order to confirm the presence of phosphorylated LASV Z protein, 5×10^5 HEK293T cells per well were seeded in six-well plates and then transfected 24 h later with 2 μg of the corresponding Z protein plasmids using 8 μg of 1 mg/mL polyethyleneinimine. Two days after transfection, the cells were treated with 8.8 mM hydrogen peroxide, or water as a control, for 20 min (min) for phosphotyrosine detection. The cells were then lysed with 1x Triton lysis buffer containing both protease and phosphatase inhibitor cocktails. SBP-tagged Z was affinity purified by incubating with streptavidin-coated magnetic beads for 2 h, followed by elution in 2x Laemmli sample buffer (125 mM Tris-HCl, 20% glycerol, 4% sodium dodecyl sulfate, and 0.02% bromophenol blue) with 5% 2-mercaptoethanol by heating at 100 °C for 10 min. The purified samples or cell input prepared in Laemmli sample buffer were separated by electrophoresis using NuPAGE 4–12% Bis-Tris gels (Thermo Fisher Scientific) with MES buffer (B000202, Thermo Fisher Scientific). Western blotting was carried out using nitrocellulose iBlot 2 gel transfer stacks (IB23001, Thermo Fisher Scientific) and the Invitrogen iBlot 2 transfer apparatus. Membranes for phosphotyrosine detection were blocked for 1 h in protein-free blocking buffer (37572, Thermo Fisher Scientific), and then a mouse anti-phosphotyrosine antibody (clone 4G10, Millipore) diluted (0.2 μg/mL) in protein-free blocking buffer was added to the membrane and incubated overnight at room temperature. The membrane was washed five times with Tris-buffered saline containing 0.1% Tween 20 (BP337, Fisher Scientific, Pittsburgh, PA, USA) (TBST), incubated for 1 h with goat anti-mouse 800 secondary antibody (926-32210, Licor, Lincoln, NE, USA) diluted 1:20,000 in 5% milk, 0.2% Tween 20 (BP337, Fisher Scientific), and 0.02% sodium dodecyl sulfate in phosphate buffered saline (PBS), and then imaged using a Licor Odyssey CLx imaging system. Immunoblotting for the Z protein was conducted by incubating the membrane with an anti-SBP tag antibody (MAB10764, Millipore, Billerica, MA, USA) diluted 1:10,000 and an anti-mouse 800 secondary antibody (926-32210, Licor) diluted 1:3000 in iBind fluorescent detection solution (SLF2019, Thermo Fisher Scientific) in an iBind Flex western device.

3.4. *Virus-Like Particle Release Assay*

To measure VLP release, 2×10^5 HEK293T cells per well were seeded in 12-well plates and then transfected 24 h later with 0.8 μg of the designated SBP-tagged LASV Z protein-expressing plasmids, using 3.2 μg of polyethyleneinimine. One day later, the VLP-containing cell culture media was collected, clarified by centrifugation, and then mixed with 10x Triton lysis buffer with a protease inhibitor cocktail to a final concentration of 1x. The cells were scraped into phosphate-buffered saline, pelleted by centrifugation, and then lysed with 1x Triton lysis buffer containing a protease inhibitor cocktail. The samples were subjected to SDS-PAGE and western blotting as described above. The SBP-tagged Z protein was detected using an anti-SBP tag antibody (MAB10764, Millipore), diluted 1:10,000 in 5% nonfat milk and 0.2% Tween 20 in PBS, and the anti-mouse 800 secondary antibody

(926-32210, Licor), diluted 1:20,000 in 5% nonfat milk, 0.02% sodium dodecyl sulfate, and 0.2% Tween 20 in PBS. In order to determine the percent VLP release, the value of each Z protein band on a particular blot was first divided by the sum of the values of all the Z protein bands on that particular blot (normalization by summation as described in [89]). This normalized Z protein quantity in VLPs was divided by the normalized Z quantity in cells for each mutant, and these values were then normalized to the corresponding quotient of Z WT, as described previously [40]. A one-way ANOVA with Holm–Sidak's test for multiple comparisons in GraphPad Prism software was used to analyze differences in VLP release.

Supplementary Materials: The following are available online at http://www.mdpi.com/2076-0817/7/4/97/s1. Figure S1: Mass spectra for identification of the Y97 and S98 phosphorylation sites in LASV Z, Figure S2: Mass spectra for identification of the S18 phosphorylation site in LASV Z.

Author Contributions: Conceptualization, C.M.Z., B.A.B., J.B.; Funding Acquisition, B.A.B. and J.B.; Investigation, C.M.Z., P.E., and M.E.W.; Project Administration, B.A.B. and J.B.; Visualization, C.M.Z., I.M., M.E.W., and B.A.B., and Writing—original draft preparation and review and editing, C.M.Z., E.A.B., B.A.B., and J.B.

Acknowledgments: The authors gratefully acknowledge NIH grants T32 AI055402 and T32 HL076122 (C.M.Z.), R21 AI088059 (J.B.), 3R41AI132047-01S1 (E.B.), and P20RR021905 and P30GM118228 (Immunobiology and Infectious Disease COBRE) (J.B.). Support for mass spectrometry analysis was provided by the Vermont Genetics Network through NIH grant 8P20GM103449 from the INBRE program and of the NIGMS.

Conflicts of Interest: The authors declare no conflicts of interest. The funding sponsors had no role in the design of the study; in the collection, analyses, or interpretation of data; in the writing of the manuscript, and in the decision to publish the results.

References

1. Charrel, R.N.; Lamballerie, X.D. Arenaviruses other than lassa virus. *Antivir. Res.* **2003**, *57*, 89–100. [CrossRef]
2. Monath, T.P.; Newhouse, V.F.; Kemp, G.E.; Setzer, H.W.; Cacciapuoti, A. Lassa virus isolation from mastomys natalensis rodents during an epidemic in sierra leone. *Science* **1974**, *185*, 263–265. [CrossRef] [PubMed]
3. Lecompte, E.; Fichet-Calvet, E.; Daffis, S.; Koulemou, K.; Sylla, O.; Kourouma, F.; Dore, A.; Soropogui, B.; Aniskin, V.; Allali, B.; et al. Mastomys natalensis and lassa fever, west africa. *Emerg. Infect. Dis.* **2006**, *12*, 1971–1974. [CrossRef] [PubMed]
4. Olayemi, A.; Cadar, D.; Magassouba, N.F.; Obadare, A.; Kourouma, F.; Oyeyiola, A.; Fasogbon, S.; Igbokwe, J.; Rieger, T.; Bockholt, S.; et al. New hosts of the lassa virus. *Sci. Rep.* **2016**, *6*, 25280. [CrossRef] [PubMed]
5. McCormick, J.B.; King, I.J.; Webb, P.A.; Scribner, C.L.; Craven, R.B.; Johnson, K.M.; Elliott, L.H.; Belmont-Williams, R. Lassa fever. *N. Engl. J. Med.* **1986**, *314*, 20–26. [CrossRef]
6. Bonwitt, J.; Kelly, A.H.; Ansumana, R.; Agbla, S.; Sahr, F.; Saez, A.M.; Borchert, M.; Kock, R.; Fichet-Calvet, E. Rat-atouille: A mixed method study to characterize rodent hunting and consumption in the context of lassa fever. *Ecohealth* **2016**, *13*, 234–247. [CrossRef] [PubMed]
7. Monath, T.P. Lassa fever: Review of epidemiology and epizootiology. *Bull. World Health Organ.* **1975**, *52*, 577–592.
8. McCormick, J.B.; Webb, P.A.; Krebs, J.W.; Johnson, K.M.; Smith, E.S. A prospective study of the epidemiology and ecology of lassa fever. *J. Infect. Dis.* **1987**, *155*, 437–444. [CrossRef] [PubMed]
9. Frame, J.D.; Baldwin, J.M.; Gocke, D.J.; Troup, J.M. Lassa fever, a new virus disease of man from west africa: I. Clinical description and pathological findings. *Am. J. Trop. Med. Hyg.* **1970**, *19*, 670–676. [CrossRef]
10. Fisher-Hoch, S.P.; Tomori, O.; Nasidi, A.; Perez-Oronoz, G.I.; Fakile, Y.; Hutwagner, L.; McCormick, J.B. Review of cases of nosocomial lassa fever in nigeria: The high price of poor medical practice. *Br. Med. J.* **1995**, *311*, 857–859. [CrossRef]
11. Ajayi, N.A.; Nwigwe, C.G.; Azuogu, B.N.; Onyire, B.N.; Nwonwu, E.U.; Ogbonnaya, L.U.; Onwe, F.I.; Ekaete, T.; Günther, S.; Ukwaja, K.N. Containing a lassa fever epidemic in a resource-limited setting: Outbreak description and lessons learned from abakaliki, nigeria (January–March 2012). *Int. J. Infect. Dis.* **2013**, *17*, e1011–e1016. [CrossRef]
12. Shaffer, J.G.; Grant, D.S.; Schieffelin, J.S.; Boisen, M.L.; Goba, A.; Hartnett, J.N.; Levy, D.C.; Yenni, R.E.; Moses, L.M.; Fullah, M.; et al. Lassa fever in post-conflict sierra leone. *PLOS Negl. Trop. Dis.* **2014**, *8*, e2748. [CrossRef]

13. Price, M.E.; Fisher-Hoch, S.P.; Craven, R.B.; McCormick, J.B. A prospective study of maternal and fetal outcome in acute lassa fever infection during pregnancy. *Br. Med. J.* **1988**, *297*, 584–587. [CrossRef]
14. Cummins, D.; McCormick, J.B.; Bennett, D.; Samba, J.A.; Farrar, B.; Machin, S.J.; Fisher-Hoch, S.P. Acute sensorineural deafness in lassa fever. *JAMA* **1990**, *264*, 2093–2096. [CrossRef] [PubMed]
15. Clegg, J.C.S.; Wilson, S.M.; Oram, J.D. Nucleotide sequence of the s rna of lassa virus (nigerian strain) and comparative analysis of arenavirus gene products. *Virus Res.* **1991**, *18*, 151–164. [CrossRef]
16. Cao, W.; Henry, M.D.; Borrow, P.; Yamada, H.; Elder, J.H.; Ravkov, E.V.; Nichol, S.T.; Compans, R.W.; Campbell, K.P.; Oldstone, M.B.A. Identification of α-dystroglycan as a receptor for lymphocytic choriomeningitis virus and lassa fever virus. *Science* **1998**, *282*, 2079–2081. [CrossRef] [PubMed]
17. Kunz, S. Receptor binding and cell entry of old world arenaviruses reveal novel aspects of virus-host interaction. *Virology* **2009**, *387*, 245–249. [CrossRef]
18. Klewitz, C.; Klenk, H.-D.; ter Meulen, J. Amino acids from both n-terminal hydrophobic regions of the lassa virus envelope glycoprotein gp-2 are critical for ph-dependent membrane fusion and infectivity. *J. Gen. Virol.* **2007**, *88*, 2320–2328. [CrossRef]
19. Lee, K.J.; Novella, I.S.; Teng, M.N.; Oldstone, M.B.A.; de la Torre, J.C. Np and l proteins of lymphocytic choriomeningitis virus (lcmv) are sufficient for efficient transcription and replication of lcmv genomic RNA analogs. *J. Virol.* **2000**, *74*, 3470–3477. [CrossRef]
20. Lopez, N.; Jacamo, R.; Franze-Fernandez, M.T. Transcription and rna replication of tacaribe virus genome and antigenome analogs require n and l proteins: Z protein is an inhibitor of these processes. *J. Virol.* **2001**, *75*, 12241–12251. [CrossRef]
21. Djavani, M.; Lukashevich, I.S.; Sanchez, A.; Nichol, S.T.; Salvato, M.S. Completion of the lassa fever virus sequence and identification of a ring finger open reading frame at the l rna 5′ end. *Virology* **1997**, *235*, 414–418. [CrossRef] [PubMed]
22. Lukashevich, I.S.; Djavani, M.; Shapiro, K.; Sanchez, A.; Ravkov, E.; Nichol, S.T.; Salvato, M.S. The lassa fever virus l gene: Nucleotide sequence, comparison, and precipitation of a predicted 250 kda protein with monospecific antiserum. *J. Gen. Virol.* **1997**, *78*, 547–551. [CrossRef]
23. Strecker, T.; Eichler, R.; Meulen, J.t.; Weissenhorn, W.; Dieter Klenk, H.; Garten, W.; Lenz, O. Lassa virus z protein is a matrix protein sufficient for the release of virus-like particles. *J. Virol.* **2003**, *77*, 10700–10705. [CrossRef] [PubMed]
24. Fehling, S.; Lennartz, F.; Strecker, T. Multifunctional nature of the arenavirus ring finger protein z. *Viruses* **2012**, *4*, 2973–3011. [CrossRef] [PubMed]
25. Xing, J.; Ly, H.; Liang, Y. The z proteins of pathogenic but not nonpathogenic arenaviruses inhibit rig-i-like receptor-dependent interferon production. *J. Virol.* **2015**, *89*, 2944–2955. [CrossRef] [PubMed]
26. Cornu, T.I.; de la Torre, J.C. Ring finger z protein of lymphocytic choriomeningitis virus (lcmv) inhibits transcription and rna replication of an lcmv s-segment minigenome. *J. Virol.* **2001**, *75*, 9415–9426. [CrossRef] [PubMed]
27. Jacamo, R.; Lopez, N.; Wilda, M.; Franze-Fernández, M.T. Tacaribe virus z protein interacts with the l polymerase protein to inhibit viral rna synthesis. *J Virol* **2003**, *77*. [CrossRef]
28. Kranzusch, P.J.; Whelan, S.P.J. Arenavirus z protein controls viral rna synthesis by locking a polymerase–promoter complex. Kranzusch, P.J.; Whelan, S.P.J. Arenavirus z protein controls viral rna synthesis by locking a polymerase–promoter complex. *Proc. Natl. Acad. Sci. USA* **2011**, *108*, 19743–19748. [CrossRef]
29. Schlie, K.; Maisa, A.; Freiberg, F.; Groseth, A.; Strecker, T.; Garten, W. Viral protein determinants of lassa virus entry and release from polarized epithelial cells. *J. Virol.* **2010**, *84*, 3178–3188. [CrossRef]
30. Capul, A.A.; Perez, M.; Burke, E.; Kunz, S.; Buchmeier, M.J.; de la Torre, J.C. Arenavirus z-glycoprotein association requires z myristoylation but not functional ring or late domains. *J. Virol.* **2007**, *81*, 9451–9460. [CrossRef]
31. Eichler, R.; Strecker, T.; Kolesnikova, L.; ter Meulen, J.; Weissenhorn, W.; Becker, S.; Klenk, H.D.; Garten, W.; Lenz, O. Characterization of the lassa virus matrix protein z: Electron microscopic study of virus-like particles and interaction with the nucleoprotein (np). *Virus Res.* **2004**, *100*, 249–255. [CrossRef] [PubMed]
32. Perez, M.; Craven, R.C.; de la Torre, J.C. The small ring finger protein z drives arenavirus budding: Implications for antiviral strategies. *Proc. Natl. Acad. Sci. USA* **2003**, *100*, 12978–12983. [CrossRef] [PubMed]

33. Zaza, A.D.; Herbreteau, C.H.; Peyrefitte, C.N.; Emonet, S.F. Mammarenaviruses deleted from their z gene are replicative and produce an infectious progeny in bhk-21 cells. *Virology* **2018**, *518*, 34–44. [CrossRef] [PubMed]
34. Strecker, T.; Maisa, A.; Daffis, S.; Eichler, R.; Lenz, O.; Garten, W. The role of myristoylation in the membrane association of the lassa virus matrix protein z. *Virol. J.* **2006**, *3*, 93. [CrossRef] [PubMed]
35. Perez, M.; Greenwald, D.L.; de La Torre, J.C. Myristoylation of the ring finger z protein is essential for arenavirus budding. *J. Virol.* **2004**, *78*, 11443–11448. [CrossRef] [PubMed]
36. Votteler, J.; Sundquist, W.I. Virus budding and the escrt pathway. *Cell Host Microbe* **2013**, *14*, 232–241. [CrossRef] [PubMed]
37. Wang, J.; Danzy, S.; Kumar, N.; Ly, H.; Liang, Y. Biological roles and functional mechanisms of arenavirus z protein in viral replication. *J. Virol.* **2012**, *86*, 9794–9801. [CrossRef]
38. Urata, S.; Noda, T.; Kawaoka, Y.; Yokosawa, H.; Yasuda, J. Cellular factors required for lassa virus budding. *J. Virol.* **2006**, *80*, 4191–4195. [CrossRef]
39. Han, Z.; Lu, J.; Liu, Y.; Davis, B.; Lee, M.S.; Olson, M.A.; Ruthel, G.; Freedman, B.D.; Schnell, M.J.; Wrobel, J.E.; et al. Small-molecule probes targeting the viral ppxy-host nedd4 interface block egress of a broad range of rna viruses. *J Virol* **2014**, *88*. [CrossRef]
40. Ziegler, C.M.; Eisenhauer, P.; Bruce, E.A.; Weir, M.E.; King, B.R.; Klaus, J.P.; Krementsov, D.N.; Shirley, D.J.; Ballif, B.A.; Botten, J. The lymphocytic choriomeningitis virus matrix protein ppxy late domain drives the production of defective interfering particles. *PLoS Pathog* **2016**, *12*, e1005501. [CrossRef]
41. Nishi, H.; Shaytan, A.; Panchenko, A.R. Physicochemical mechanisms of protein regulation by phosphorylation. *Front. Genet.* **2014**, *5*, 270. [CrossRef] [PubMed]
42. Keck, F.; Ataey, P.; Amaya, M.; Bailey, C.; Narayanan, A. Phosphorylation of single stranded rna virus proteins and potential for novel therapeutic strategies. *Viruses* **2015**, *7*, 5257–5273. [CrossRef] [PubMed]
43. Schwartz, D.; Church, G.M. Collection and motif-based prediction of phosphorylation sites in human viruses. *Sci. Signal.* **2010**, *3*, rs2. [CrossRef] [PubMed]
44. Bretaña, N.A.; Lu, C.-T.; Chiang, C.-Y.; Su, M.-G.; Huang, K.-Y.; Lee, T.-Y.; Weng, S.-L. Identifying protein phosphorylation sites with kinase substrate specificity on human viruses. *PLoS ONE* **2012**, *7*, e40694. [CrossRef] [PubMed]
45. Keating, J.A.; Striker, R. Phosphorylation events during viral infections provide potential therapeutic targets. *Rev. Med. Virol.* **2012**, *22*, 166–181. [CrossRef] [PubMed]
46. García, M.; Cooper, A.; Shi, W.; Bornmann, W.; Carrion, R.; Kalman, D.; Nabel, G.J. Productive replication of ebola virus is regulated by the c-abl1 tyrosine kinase. *Sci. Transl. Med.* **2012**, *4*, 123ra124. [CrossRef] [PubMed]
47. Kolesnikova, L.; Mittler, E.; Schudt, G.; Shams-Eldin, H.; Becker, S. Phosphorylation of marburg virus matrix protein vp40 triggers assembly of nucleocapsids with the viral envelope at the plasma membrane. *Cell. Microbiol.* **2012**, *14*, 182–197. [CrossRef]
48. Bajorek, M.; Caly, L.; Tran, K.C.; Maertens, G.N.; Tripp, R.A.; Bacharach, E.; Teng, M.N.; Ghildyal, R.; Jans, D.A. The thr205 phosphorylation site within respiratory syncytial virus matrix (m) protein modulates m oligomerization and virus production. *J. Virol.* **2014**. [CrossRef]
49. Pei, Z.; Harrison, M.S.; Schmitt, A.P. Parainfluenza virus 5 m protein interaction with host protein 14-3-3 negatively affects virus particle formation. *J. Virol.* **2011**, *85*, 2050–2059. [CrossRef]
50. Hemonnot, B.; Mollé, D.; Bardy, M.; Gay, B.; Laune, D.; Devaux, C.; Briant, L. Phosphorylation of the htlv-1 matrix l-domain-containing protein by virus-associated erk-2 kinase. *Virology* **2006**, *349*, 430–439. [CrossRef]
51. Ziegler, C.M.; Eisenhauer, P.; Bruce, E.A.; Beganovic, V.; King, B.R.; Weir, M.E.; Ballif, B.A.; Botten, J. A novel phosphoserine motif in the lcmv matrix protein z regulates the release of infectious virus and defective interfering particles. *J. Gen. Virol.* **2016**, *97*, 2084–2089. [CrossRef] [PubMed]
52. Volpon, L.; Osborne, M.J.; Capul, A.A.; de la Torre, J.C.; Borden, K.L.B. Structural characterization of the z ring-eif4e complex reveals a distinct mode of control for eif4e. *Proc. Natl. Acad. Sci. USA* **2010**, *107*, 5441–5446. [CrossRef] [PubMed]
53. Salvato, M.S.; Schweighofer, K.J.; Burns, J.; Shimomaye, E.M. Biochemical and immunological evidence that the 11 kda zinc-binding protein of lymphocytic choriomeningitis virus is a structural component of the virus. *Virus Res.* **1992**, *22*, 185–198. [CrossRef]
54. Salvato, M.S.; Shimomaye, E.M. The completed sequence of lymphocytic choriomeningitis virus reveals a unique rna structure and a gene for a zinc finger protein. *Virology* **1989**, *173*, 1–10. [CrossRef]

55. Hastie, K.M.; Zandonatti, M.; Liu, T.; Li, S.; Woods, V.L.; Saphire, E.O. Crystal structure of the oligomeric form of lassa virus matrix protein z. *J. Virol.* **2016**, *90*, 4556–4562. [CrossRef] [PubMed]
56. Volpon, L.; Osborne, M.J.; Borden, K.L.B. Nmr assignment of the arenaviral protein z from lassa fever virus. *Biomol. NMR Assign.* **2008**, *2*, 81–84. [CrossRef]
57. May, E.R.; Armen, R.S.; Mannan, A.M.; Brooks, C.L. The flexible c-terminal arm of the lassa arenavirus z-protein mediates interactions with multiple binding partners. *Proteins* **2010**, *78*, 2251–2264. [CrossRef]
58. Capul, A.A.; de la Torre, J.C.; Buchmeier, M.J. Conserved residues in lassa fever virus z protein modulate viral infectivity at the level of the ribonucleoprotein. *J. Virol.* **2011**, *85*, 3172–3178. [CrossRef]
59. Xing, J.; Chai, Z.; Ly, H.; Liang, Y. Differential inhibition of macrophage activation by lymphocytic choriomeningitis virus and pichinde virus is mediated by the z protein n-terminal domain. *J. Virol.* **2015**, *89*, 12513–12517. [CrossRef]
60. Li, W.; Cowley, A.; Uludag, M.; Gur, T.; McWilliam, H.; Squizzato, S.; Park, Y.M.; Buso, N.; Lopez, R. The embl-ebi bioinformatics web and programmatic tools framework. *Nucleic Acids Res.* **2015**, *43*, W580–W584. [CrossRef]
61. Manning, J.T.; Forrester, N.; Paessler, S. Lassa virus isolates from mali and the ivory coast represent an emerging fifth lineage. *Front. Microbiol.* **2015**, *6*, 1037. [CrossRef] [PubMed]
62. Bowen, M.D.; Rollin, P.E.; Ksiazek, T.G.; Hustad, H.L.; Bausch, D.G.; Demby, A.H.; Bajani, M.D.; Peters, C.J.; Nichol, S.T. Genetic diversity among lassa virus strains. *J. Virol.* **2000**, *74*, 6992–7004. [CrossRef] [PubMed]
63. Shannon, L.M.W.; Thomas, S.; Daniel, C.; Hans-Peter, D.; Kelly, F.; Ketan, P.; Shelley, M.B.; William, G.D.; John, D.K.; Pierre, E.R.; et al. New lineage of lassa virus, togo, 2016. *Emerg. Infect. Dis. J.* **2018**, *24*, 599.
64. Oloniniyi, O.K.; Unigwe, U.S.; Okada, S.; Kimura, M.; Koyano, S.; Miyazaki, Y.; Iroezindu, M.O.; Ajayi, N.A.; Chukwubike, C.M.; Chika-Igwenyi, N.M.; et al. Genetic characterization of lassa virus strains isolated from 2012 to 2016 in southeastern nigeria. *PLOS Negl. Trop. Dis.* **2018**, *12*, e0006971. [CrossRef] [PubMed]
65. Verdecia, M.A.; Bowman, M.E.; Lu, K.P.; Hunter, T.; Noel, J.P. Structural basis for phosphoserine-proline recognition by group iv ww domains. *Nat. Struct. Biol.* **2000**, *7*, 639. [CrossRef] [PubMed]
66. Smerdon, S.J.; Yaffe, M.B. Chapter 72-recognition of phospho-serine/threonine phosphorylated proteins by phospho-serine/threonine-binding domains. In *Handbook of Cell Signaling*, 2nd ed.; Bradshaw, R.A., Dennis, E.A., Eds.; Academic Press: San Diego, CA, USA, 2010; pp. 539–550.
67. Liou, Y.-C.; Zhou, X.Z.; Lu, K.P. Prolyl isomerase pin1 as a molecular switch to determine the fate of phosphoproteins. *Trends Biochem. Sci.* **2011**, *36*, 501–514. [CrossRef] [PubMed]
68. Pang, R.; Lee, T.K.W.; Poon, R.T.P.; Fan, S.T.; Wong, K.B.; Kwong, Y.L.; Tse, E. Pin1 interacts with a specific serine-proline motif of hepatitis b virus x-protein to enhance hepatocarcinogenesis. *Gastroenterology* **2007**, *132*, 1088–1103. [CrossRef]
69. Jeong, S.-J.; Ryo, A.; Yamamoto, N. The prolyl isomerase pin1 stabilizes the human t-cell leukemia virus type 1 (htlv-1) tax oncoprotein and promotes malignant transformation. *Biochem. Biophys. Res. Commun.* **2009**, *381*, 294–299. [CrossRef]
70. Peloponese, J.-M.; Yasunaga, J.; Kinjo, T.; Watashi, K.; Jeang, K.-T. Peptidylproline cis-trans-isomerase pin1 interacts with human t-cell leukemia virus type 1 tax and modulates its activation of nf-κb. *J. Virol.* **2009**, *83*, 3238–3248. [CrossRef]
71. Misumi, S.; Inoue, M.; Dochi, T.; Kishimoto, N.; Hasegawa, N.; Takamune, N.; Shoji, S. Uncoating of human immunodeficiency virus type 1 requires prolyl isomerase pin1. *J. Biol. Chem.* **2010**, *285*, 25185–25195. [CrossRef]
72. Dochi, T.; Nakano, T.; Inoue, M.; Takamune, N.; Shoji, S.; Sano, K.; Misumi, S. Phosphorylation of human immunodeficiency virus type 1 capsid protein at serine 16, required for peptidyl-prolyl isomerase-dependent uncoating, is mediated by virion-incorporated extracellular signal-regulated kinase 2. *J. Gen. Virol.* **2014**, *95*, 1156–1166. [CrossRef] [PubMed]
73. Manganaro, L.; Lusic, M.; Gutierrez, M.I.; Cereseto, A.; Del Sal, G.; Giacca, M. Concerted action of cellular jnk and pin1 restricts hiv-1 genome integration to activated cd4+ t lymphocytes. *Nat. Med.* **2010**, *16*, 329. [CrossRef] [PubMed]
74. Narita, Y.; Murata, T.; Ryo, A.; Kawashima, D.; Sugimoto, A.; Kanda, T.; Kimura, H.; Tsurumi, T. Pin1 interacts with the epstein-barr virus DNA polymerase catalytic subunit and regulates viral DNA replication. *J. Virol.* **2013**, *87*, 2120–2127. [CrossRef]

75. Guito, J.; Gavina, A.; Palmeri, D.; Lukac, D.M. The cellular peptidyl-prolyl cis/trans isomerase pin1 regulates reactivation of kaposi's sarcoma-associated herpesvirus from latency. *J. Virol.* **2014**, *88*, 547–558. [CrossRef]
76. Denu, J.M.; Tanner, K.G. Specific and reversible inactivation of protein tyrosine phosphatases by hydrogen peroxide: Evidence for a sulfenic acid intermediate and implications for redox regulation. *Biochemistry* **1998**, *37*, 5633–5642. [CrossRef] [PubMed]
77. Dephoure, N.; Gould, K.L.; Gygi, S.P.; Kellogg, D.R.; Drubin, D.G. Mapping and analysis of phosphorylation sites: A quick guide for cell biologists. *Mol. Biol. Cell* **2013**, *24*, 535–542. [CrossRef] [PubMed]
78. Huang, A.S.; Baltimore, D. Defective viral particles and viral disease processes. *Nature* **1970**, *226*, 325–327. [CrossRef]
79. Dutko, F.J.; Pfau, C.J. Arenavirus defective interfering particles mask the cell-killing potential of standard virus. *J. Gen. Virol.* **1978**, *38*, 195–208. [CrossRef]
80. Carnec, X.; Baize, S.; Reynard, S.; Diancourt, L.; Caro, V.; Tordo, N.; Bouloy, M. Lassa virus nucleoprotein mutants generated by reverse genetics induce a robust type i interferon response in human dendritic cells and macrophages. *J. Virol.* **2011**, *85*, 12093–12097. [CrossRef]
81. Popescu, M.; Schaefer, H.; Lehmann-Grube, F. Homologous interference of lymphocytic choriomeningitis virus: Detection and measurement of interference focus-forming units. *J. Virol.* **1976**, *20*, 1–8.
82. Welsh, R.M.; Pfau, C.J. Determinants of lymphocytic choriomeningitis interference. *J. Gen. Virol.* **1972**, *14*, 177–187. [CrossRef] [PubMed]
83. Chesarino, N.M.; McMichael, T.M.; Hach, J.C.; Yount, J.S. Phosphorylation of the antiviral protein interferon-inducible transmembrane protein 3 (ifitm3) dually regulates its endocytosis and ubiquitination. *J. Biol. Chem.* **2014**, *289*, 11986–11992. [CrossRef] [PubMed]
84. Sotgia, F.; Lee, H.; Bedford, M.T.; Petrucci, T.; Sudol, M.; Lisanti, M.P. Tyrosine phosphorylation of β-dystroglycan at its ww domain binding motif, ppxy, recruits sh2 domain containing proteins. *Biochemistry* **2001**, *40*, 14585–14592. [CrossRef] [PubMed]
85. Chesarino, N.M.; McMichael, T.M.; Yount, J.S. E3 ubiquitin ligase nedd4 promotes influenza virus infection by decreasing levels of the antiviral protein ifitm3. *PLOS Pathogens* **2015**, *11*, e1005095. [CrossRef] [PubMed]
86. Cornillez-Ty, C.T.; Liao, L.; Yates, J.R.; Kuhn, P.; Buchmeier, M.J. Severe acute respiratory syndrome coronavirus nonstructural protein 2 interacts with a host protein complex involved in mitochondrial biogenesis and intracellular signaling. *J. Virol.* **2009**, *83*, 10314–10318. [CrossRef] [PubMed]
87. Klaus, J.P.; Eisenhauer, P.; Russo, J.; Mason, A.B.; Do, D.; King, B.; Taatjes, D.; Cornillez-Ty, C.; Boyson, J.E.; Thali, M.; et al. The intracellular cargo receptor ergic-53 is required for the production of infectious arenavirus, coronavirus, and filovirus particles. *Cell Host Microbe* **2013**, *14*, 522–534. [CrossRef] [PubMed]
88. Ziegler, C.M.; Eisenhauer, P.; Kelly, J.A.; Dang, L.N.; Beganovic, V.; Bruce, E.A.; King, B.R.; Shirley, D.J.; Weir, M.E.; Ballif, B.A.; et al. A proteomics survey of junín virus interactions with human proteins reveals host factors required for arenavirus replication. *J. Virol.* **2018**, *92*, e01565-17. [CrossRef]
89. Degasperi, A.; Birtwistle, M.R.; Volinsky, N.; Rauch, J.; Kolch, W.; Kholodenko, B.N. Evaluating strategies to normalise biological replicates of western blot data. *PLoS ONE* **2014**, *9*, e87293. [CrossRef]

pathogens

MDPI

Review

Improving the Breadth of the Host's Immune Response to Lassa Virus

Juan Carlos Zapata *, Sandra Medina-Moreno, Camila Guzmán-Cardozo and Maria S. Salvato

Institute of Human Virology, School of Medicine, University of Maryland, Baltimore, MD 21201, USA; smmoreno@ihv.umaryland.edu (S.M.-M.); mcguzmanc13@gmail.com (C.G.-C.); MSalvato@ihv.umaryland.edu (M.S.S.)

* Correspondence: jczapata@ihv.umaryland.edu; Tel.: +1-443-416-9506

Received: 21 September 2018; Accepted: 24 October 2018; Published: 28 October 2018

Abstract: In 2017, the global Coalition for Epidemic Preparedness (CEPI) declared Lassa virus disease to be one of the world's foremost biothreats. In January 2018, World Health Organization experts met to address the Lassa biothreat. It was commonly recognized that the diversity of Lassa virus (LASV) isolated from West African patient samples was far greater than that of the Ebola isolates from the West African epidemic of 2013–2016. Thus, vaccines produced against Lassa virus disease face the added challenge that they must be broadly-protective against a wide variety of LASV. In this review, we discuss what is known about the immune response to Lassa infection. We also discuss the approaches used to make broadly-protective influenza vaccines and how they could be applied to developing broad vaccine coverage against LASV disease. Recent advances in AIDS research are also potentially applicable to the design of broadly-protective medical countermeasures against LASV disease.

Keywords: Lassa virus disease (LVD); vaccine breadth; mimicry; B cell anergy; conserved antigens; Fc-gamma receptors; conformational antigens; broadly-neutralizing antibodies; focused immunity; dominant and subdominant epitopes; cross-restriction

---

1. Introduction

Lassa virus (LASV) is a zoonotic pathogen endemic to West Africa. Annual outbreaks occur primarily during the dry season amongst the rural population [1]. In December 2013, West Africa experienced an outbreak of Ebola virus that quickly grew into an epidemic, revealing that much of this part of the world was unprepared to handle such a disaster. The Ebola epidemic was a more terrifying version of the annual Lassa disease outbreaks, and was characterized by high person-to-person transmission, the deaths of medical personnel, popular hysteria and occasional transmission outside West Africa [2]. It became clear that the unchecked spread of such infections could endanger the rest of the world.

In 2017, the global Coalition for Epidemic Preparedness (CEPI) declared Lassa virus disease to be one of the world's foremost biothreats [3]. In January 2018, the World Health Organization (WHO) convened a "Lassa Roadmap" panel lead by Mike Osterholm, an epidemiologist and expert in biosecurity [4]. As the panel considered the technical obstacles to Lassa vaccine production, one of the more important obstacles was "breadth of vaccine protection". Breadth refers to the variety of infections suppressed by one vaccine. If the vaccine is broadly protective, it might shield vaccinees from all of the genetically diverse Lassa lineages identified in patient samples [5]. Sequencing studies of blood from infected West African patients showed an almost 50-fold greater variation of LASV isolates than of Ebola virus isolates [6,7]. This means that a Lassa vaccine needs to be more broadly protective than an Ebola vaccine because it needs to cover a greater genetic variation. This variation is presumably due to the fact that most of the Lassa patients are infected directly through the rodent reservoir, whereas most Ebola patients are infected by contact with other human patients. Hence, the high variation of Lassa outbreaks is due to multiple introductions from the rodents and not to any changes in viral mutation rate. Another contributing factor may be that LASV replication in culture generates 10–1000-fold fewer virus particles per infectious particle than Ebola virus Zaire or Sudan isolates [8]. This means Ebola virus produces an excess of viral products and only a few of them assemble to become infectious particles.

Vaccine cross-protection reflects the genetic diversity covered by a vaccine. If a Lassa vaccine is "narrowly protective", it will only protect against one or two Lassa lineages: two closely-related lineages differ in 5–7% of their nucleotide sequence. If the vaccine is more broadly protective, it could protect against all Lassa lineages (the most divergent LASV lineages differ by as much as 27% of their nucleotides) [9]. If the vaccine is even broader, it should protect against other arenavirus species. The genetic diversity between LASV species and a closely related Old World arenavirus species such as LCMV ranges 30–50% difference between their nucleotide sequences [9].

The last 50 years of LASV research shed some light on its pathogenesis and effects on the host immune response. During the early innate response, LASV infection seems to affect dendritic cell function, resulting in poor antigen-presentation, partial immunosuppression and unchecked virus replication [10–12]. In monkeys and in Lassa-infected people, neutralizing antibodies are slow to develop, partially due to glycans on the viral envelope (GP) that mimic self-glycans and anergize the B cell response [13].

Several LASV vaccine candidates have demonstrated efficacy in animal models. A live attenuated MOP/LAS reassortant vaccine (clone ML29), designed by Lukashevich and further developed to pre-clinical studies in our laboratory, has shown sterilizing protection against Lassa disease in mice, guinea pigs, and non-human primates [14–18]. Additionally, this vaccine elicits immune responses to LASV glycoprotein (GP) and nucleoprotein (NP), even in primates chronically-infected with SIV [19]. In this review, we discuss the Lassa vaccine candidates that have demonstrated broad cross-protection and the key properties contributing to their breadth.

The goal of this review is to discuss possible ways to improve the immune response to LASV. In the first part, we discuss what is known about the development of immune responses to Lassa virus and the current vaccine candidates used to confer antiviral immunity, then we describe the approaches used to obtain "universal flu vaccines" and broadly protective AIDS vaccines, and how these approaches could possibly be applied to medical countermeasures against Lassa fever.

2. Clinical Manifestations and Pathogenesis of Lassa Virus Disease

LASV pathogenesis and its failure to develop strong immune responses remain a mystery. Although there is a strong correlation between the level of viremia and the disease outcome (Figure 1), the damage is not caused directly by viral-cell lysis and seems to depend on the initial host immune response [20–22]. The first symptoms are poorly differentiated from other diseases. In addition, the incubation period can be as long as two weeks. Those two situations make the initial diagnosis difficult and cause a delay in the initiation of the treatment. Twenty percent of the infected patients develop symptoms of muscle fatigue, facial edema, and sore throat, and a few of these progress to systemic disease with mucosal, conjunctival, gastrointestinal or genital bleeding. Platelet dysfunction and endothelial damage seem to play a role in the characteristic vascular leakage.

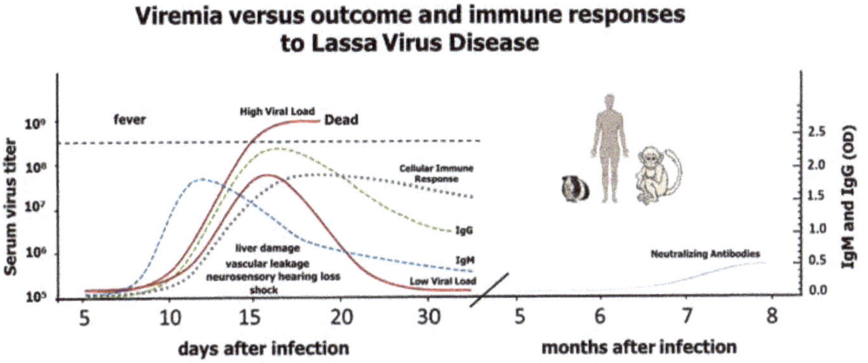

Figure 1. This is a representation of LASV viremia in relation to Lassa virus disease outcomes and immune responses to Lassa virus based on published data about rodent, non-human primate and human infections. When the immune system fails to control the virus, disease is more acute and leads to death. Those individuals with moderate viral replication (~80%) are either asymptomatic or, if they develop symptoms, they have higher possibilities to survive (low solid red line), while those patients with high viral loads suffer severe disease that can lead to death (high solid red line) [21,23]. Dotted lines represent cellular and humoral immune responses. Solid blue line represents the rise of neutralizing antibodies.

Fatal cases are associated with myocarditis, pulmonary edema, acute respiratory distress, and a hypovolemic shock; in addition, elevated plasma aminotransferases (AST and ALT), uncontrolled viremia, and high levels of IL-6 are pathognomonic for LF [22]. Massive viral replication in the liver and spleen leads to progressive hemorrhagic manifestations and increased mortality. It is common to find hepatocellular necrosis and foci of hepatocyte proliferation [24–26]. A recent description of arenavirus-induced liver pathology was characterized by hepatocytes with increased cell death, upregulated cell cycling factor p21, IFN-γ, and LASV receptor Axl-1, but aborted cell cycling. Whereas mature hepatocytes had low alpha-dystroglycan (α-DG; a LSV receptor) expression, oval cells had high expression of α-DG [27]. Coagulation disorders are not common in LF; however, when they happen, platelet counts could be normal with little disseminated intravascular coagulation, while platelet aggregation is impaired and loss of liquids [28–32]. Neuropathological manifestations include disorientation, motor and sensory abnormalities, convulsions, hiccups, and in advanced stages coma. Brain dysfunctions are associated with poor prognosis and it is not clear if they are the result of the direct effect of LASV, nonspecific metabolites, or immune-mediated effects. LASV infection is responsible for the high prevalence of hearing loss in West Africa: around 30% of LF patients develop hearing problems and 17% of LF survivors suffer permanent hearing loss [33–37].

3. Early Immune Response to Lassa Virus Infection

LF survivors are able to control viral loads early during the infection. In contrast, fatal cases show poor inflammatory responses characterized by lymphopenia, that affects all lymphocyte subpopulations, including CD4+ and CD8+ T cells, B cells, and NK cells, along with necrosis of lymphoid organs [29,38–41]. This immuno-suppressive state appears to be induced early during the infection. In vitro LASV infection of macrophages, dendritic cells (DC), and endothelial cells down-regulated the production of inflammatory mediators [10,11,42]. In vivo, antigen presenting cells (APC; macrophages (MP) and dendritic cells (DC)) are the primary targets of LASV. In monkeys, by seven days after infection, infected DC were found in a variety of tissues. MP were also infected to a lesser extent. Kupffer cells, hepatocytes, adreno-cortical cells and endothelial cells were more frequently infected in the tissues of terminal animals. In lymph nodes, LASV antigen was detected in

DC located in the marginal zone and to a lesser extent in monocytes and MP in the marginal zone and red pulp [40].

Most RNA viruses activate DC and MP while replicating due to the production of dsRNA genomic intermediates and other viral sub-products presenting pathogen molecular patterns (PAMPs), which are recognized by specialized pattern recognition receptors (PRR). LASV PAMPs activate several signaling cascades that lead to the secretion of chemokines and cytokines, including interferon (IFN) responses that inhibit virus replication and induce cellular genes involved in innate and adaptive immunity [43,44]. Although sensitive to the antiviral effects of IFN-α and IFN-γ, LASV has been shown to regulate IFN production in vitro and in vivo [10,11,42,45]. In lethally-infected animals, IFN-γ levels were moderately elevated [46] and, in human fatal cases, IFN-γ levels were increased in some individuals [47]. In macaques, IFN type I was detected very early in survivors but only in the late stages of fatal cases [38]. The inhibition of IFN by LASV affects plasmacytoid DC maturation and reduces production of cytokines and chemokines by these cells [43,48]. Another function inhibited by the block to DC maturation is their capacity to migrate to the secondary lymphoid organs, to express CCR7, and thus to activate T cells [11].

A common feature of the viral nucleoprotein (NP) of mammalian arenaviruses is its ability to prevent nuclear translocation of interferon regulatory factor 3 (IRF-3), IFN type I activation, and the downstream induction of the interferon stimulated genes (ISG) [48–51]. The anti-IFN activity of NP is located in its C-terminus that is structurally homologous to the DEDDH family of 3′-5′ exoribonucleases [52]. The NP crystal structure and its interaction with RIG-I and MDA-5 suggest that NP ribonuclease activity is able to remove viral PAMP RNA, thereby avoiding recognition by PRRs and inhibiting IFN production [52,53]. The LASV Z matrix protein also binds RIG-I and MDA-5 to inhibit type I IFN induction [54]. In contrast to NP, Z proteins of some arenaviruses do not bind RIG-I/MDA-5 and fail to inhibit IFN production [54]. The authors suggest that Z-mediated anti-IFN activity is more frequently associated with pathogenic arenaviruses. Another group, showing that the L polymerase is subject to more positive selection events (>dN/dS) during evolution than any other arenaviral gene, argues that the polymerase might be central to viral pathogenesis [55].

LASV infection of monocyte and endothelial cell cultures suppressed TNF-α and IL-8, an effect that in vivo would be predicted to inhibit inflammation and neutrophil migration [10]. In contrast, infected monocyte-derived DC showed an increase in IL-8 secretion with a reduction in the expression of co-stimulatory molecules such as CD86, CD80, and CD40. Additionally, LASV-infected DC failed to produce pro-inflammatory cytokines and to stimulate T cells [42]. Although both MP and DC are susceptible to LASV infection, immature DC supported virus replication without being destroyed or activated. Neither the infection of human DC and MP nor their stimulation with inactivated virus induced the production of TNF-α, IL-1β, IL-2, IL-6, IL-8, IL-10, IL-12p35, TGF- β, IFN-γ, or CD25 [11,42].

In line with the cell culture results, LF fatal cases see a reduction in IL-8 and IP-10 in comparison to survivors [11,42]. Similar results were seen in vivo in cynomolgus macaques [40]. IL-8 was the only cytokine that peaked in infected people who did not develop LASV disease [56]. In addition, primates and human PBMC exposed to LCMV-WE (a virus causing hemorrhagic fever) showed that virulent infection was associated with undetectable levels of TNF-α, low levels of IL-8 in plasma and inhibition of IL-8 mRNA expression [46,57].

In vitro, LASV and LCMV-WE down-regulated IL-6 and other pro-inflammatory cyto/chemokines in human MP and epithelial cells. In contrast, MOPV and LCMV-ARM strongly up-regulated pro-inflammatory responses in a TLR-2/Mal-dependent manner [58]. Meanwhile, a high level of IL-6 in plasma is a biomarker of progressing LF in humans and in primates experimentally infected with LASV or LCMV-WE. This high level of IL-6 during the last stages of severe LF could result from hepatic regeneration and may be associated with neutrophilia [22,24,38,46,59]. We speculate that the in vitro studies model the earliest events in LASV infection, whereas the IL-6 in infected macaque plasma is a late event of LASV infection; hence, severe pathology would be marked by early suppression of IL-6 and late abundance of IL-6.

Taken together, the above evidence suggests that LASV targets monocytes and DC, inhibits the initial immune response and suppresses the migration of activated cells to the primary infection site resulting in higher viral replication, greater virulence, and a delay in the induction of the acquired immune response.

4. Acquired Immunity to Lassa Virus Infection

LASV-specific IgM and IgG are detected during peak viremia, and appear unrelated to recovery from disease [20]. Primate immunization with gamma-irradiated LASV, an inactivation procedure that preserves the natural structure of antigens, induced strong antibody responses to NP and GP antigens, but failed to protect immunized animals from fatal LF [60]. Notably, NP is the earliest antigen detected by antigen-capture assays in infected individuals, most likely because it is the most abundant structural component of each virion [61]. In addition, ELISA to detect NP antibody was used in early seroprevalence studies [62]. Due to the structural importance of NP, it is likely to contribute to the breadth of the acquired immune response to LASV (see arguments in Section 6).

In cynomolgus macaques experimentally infected with LASV, the antibody titers against GP1, GP2, and NP increased more rapidly in survivors than in fatal cases [38]. Neutralizing antibodies (nAbs) in convalescing people can be detected only in low titers, several months after the initial infection and have been LASV strain-specific [23,63]. These findings suggest that the antibody response may not be responsible for the patient's recovery. However, antibodies could be playing an important role in attenuating acute infection, as suggested by its early appearance in surviving monkeys, the high seroprevalence in endemic areas without clinically overt disease, the lack of disease in infected contacts or the high mortality rate in individuals from LASV-free regions [38,56,64].

Treatment of human beings and animals with immune-antiserum showed a range of results [23,65–67]. A study testing a cocktail of human nAbs, generated in vitro from $LASV_{Josiah}$-infected individuals, was able to rescue late-stage infected macaques from death. In those experiments, viremic macaques were treated with a single dose of the cocktail at Days 6 and 8 after LASV infection leading to virus clearance and survival [68]. Although antibody cocktails of 15 mg nAb /kg macaque constitute an expensive treatment, their success is an important proof-of-concept. Recent structural studies revealed that artificially-generated nAbs recognized a metastable pre-fusion GP complex and blocked changes required for engagement with the intracellular receptor LAMP-1 and fusion with host membrane in late endosomes [69]. However, LASV infection induces predominantly non-nAbs against conserved NP and GP2 antigens and with a few exceptions these antibodies become undetectable after several months [62,70]. Seronegative survivors (approximately 18% of total within the LASV endemic areas) were not resistant to LASV re-infection but were protected from clinical LF [71].

After acute LF recovery, patients overcome the initial lymphopenia and develop a strong CD4+ immune response against NP and GP2. The NP-CD4+ response is only partially strain-specific since it cross-reacts with other LASV strains [72]. The LASV-GP2-CD4+-specific response recognizes a conserved epitope that is common in the Old World (100% similarity with LCMV) and New World arenaviruses (>90% similarity) [73]. In animal models, T cell responses are more important than B cells responses, and the CTL-mediated protection seems to rely more on CD8+ cells than on CD4+ cells [19]. In LASV-infected monkeys T-cell activation was delayed in fatal cases and in vitro stimulation of lymphocytes from those animals did not result in proliferation [38]. There were also decreases in CD20+ cells, and down-regulation of class II MHC antigens [25]. In contrast to fatal cases, survivors showed activation and proliferation after exposure to inactivated LASV, as well as an increase in circulating monocytes [38]. Similarly, ML29 immunization of marmosets increased the number of CD3+ and CD14+ cells [25].

The LASV-infection of one health care worker gave the USA Centers for Disease Control the rare opportunity to monitor blood cells during disease progression in a human patient [74]. During the acute phase, CD4 and CD8 T cells peaked in conjunction with virus clearance. During convalescence, the CD4 T cells waned while CD8 T cell activation and degranulation peaked for a second time. The patient was ultimately able to generate long-term, polyfunctional, Lassa virus-specific T cells, with approximately 66% of the CD4 T cells and 75% of the CD8 T cells expressing more than one cytokine. Taken together, these results suggest strong participation of T cell responses in protection and recovery during natural LASV infection. However, despite recent successful recoveries, the mechanism of protection remains unknown and more studies of human cases are needed to characterize the role of T cells in LF protection [15,41,70,75–77]. The evidence suggests that the inhibition of pattern recognition receptors (PRR) by LASV at the beginning of the infection, and the failure to induce early pro-inflammatory cytokines results in a temporary immunosuppression and uncontrolled virus replication. An early and strong immune response that controls virus replication is more likely to promote recovery from LASV disease.

5. A comparison of Promising Lassa Vaccine Candidates

Immunization of monkeys and guinea pigs with LCMV, MOBV, MOPV, and other non-pathogenic Old-World viruses can all confer some protection against LF disease [15,19,41,70,75,76,78] (Figure 2). Mopeia virus (MOPV), an arenavirus species found in rodents of eastern and southern Africa, serves as a naturally attenuated vaccine, protecting non-human primates from a lethal challenge with LASV [78,79]. The fact that MOPV and LASV can cross-protect, even though they belong to different species shows that broadly-protective vaccines are feasible. Knowledge that MOPV is a widespread, cross-protecting and non-pathogenic virus led to the production of at least two vaccines based on the MOPV platform (ML29 and MOP-VAC).

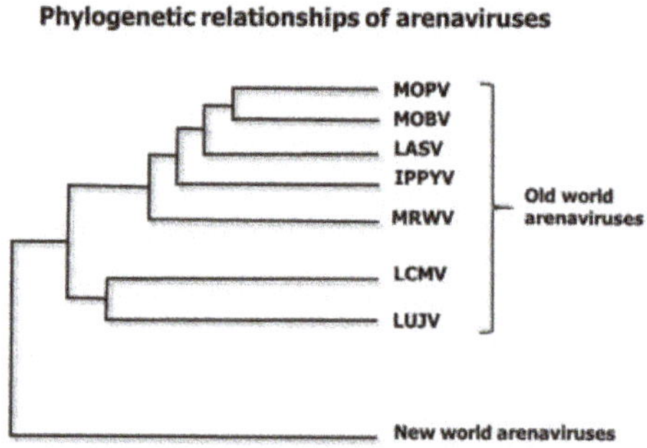

Figure 2. Phylogenetic relationships of some Old-World arenavirus species. LASV is related to several "Old World" arenaviruses. Mopeia virus AN20410 (NC_006574.1) is designated MOPV. Mobala virus (NC_007904.1) is MOBV. Lassa virus (NC_004297.1) is LASV. Ippy virus (NC_007906 is IPPYV. Merino Walk Virus (NC_023763.1) is MRWV. Lymphocytic choriomeningitis virus (NC_004291.1 is LCMV. Lujo virus (NC_012777.1) is LUJV. The family *Arenaviridae* has three genera: *Mammarenaviruses*, *Reptarenaviruses* and *Hartmaniviruses* [80]. Here, we only depict seven species of the Old-World group of the *Mammarenavirus* genus, omitting the New World *Mammarenaviruses* and the other two genera. This is a maximum clade credibility tree of the polymerase region. The tree was constructed from amino acid alignment using Bayesian MCMC method with LG model of substitution.

In this section, we compare five Lassa vaccine candidates with respect to their estimated economy of production, safety for pregnant women, breadth of protection, and capacity to confer sterilizing immunity after a lethal challenge (Table 1). Published claims and extrapolated guesses have been used for these estimates, since no pair of these vaccines has yet been put to a rigorous head-to-head comparison. Such a comparison should eventually be done for the benefit of all stakeholders.

ML29, derived from lineage IV $Lassa_{Josiah}$, is considered a broadly cross-protective Lassa vaccine because it showed sterilizing immunity in guinea pigs challenged with a distantly-related lineage

II strain of Lassa virus [5,16]. Broad cross-protection by ML29 was also observed in SIV-infected rhesus macaques given a lethal challenge with LCMV-WE. Whereas naive macaques given LCMV-WE succumbed to a LF-like febrile illness, four macaques immunized with ML29 survived for a month without increases in plasma AST or ALT (MSS unpublished, with remaining animals from [19]). This finding was consistent with the previous observation that ML29-inoculated rhesus macaques induced strong cross-reactive cell-mediated immunity to LCMV-WE [15].

The VSV-Las vaccine is a rhabdovirus vector expressing a single Lassa gene, the GPC. Guinea pigs vaccinated with VSV-Las_{Josiah} were challenged with two closely-related strains, Liberian $Lassa_{Z\text{-}132}$, and a Malian $Lassa_{SorombaR}$. Currently, there is no challenge model for LASV from lineage I $LASV_{Pinneo}$, so in these experiments all animals survived including the challenge controls, making it impossible to justify claims about cross-protection from $LASV_{Pinneo}$. Three cynomolgus macaques vaccinated with VSV-Las_{GP} and challenged with the related lineage IV strain, $Lassa_{Z\text{-}132}$, also survived. Monkey challenges with distantly-related strains such as $LASV_{Pinneo}$ were not reported. Thus, in contrast to ML29, the VSV-Las_{GP} has demonstrated only narrow protection against LASV lineages closely-related to the vaccine and has failed to demonstrate sterilizing immunity [81].

Lassa vaccine testing in guinea pigs has given misleading positive results in the past, for example a LasNP vaccine was able to protect guinea pigs but not primates [82]. Cross-protection between LCMV and LASV in guinea pigs was less effective in primates [83]. Vaccines constructed on the yellow fever vaccine platform, YF17D, were found to work well in guinea pigs but were relatively disappointing in primates. It was discovered that the YF-Las_{GP1} and YF-LAS_{GP2} vaccines were more stable than the YF-Las_{GPC} vaccine and protected 80% of guinea pigs [84,85] but failed to protect marmosets (I. Lukashevich, unpublished). We would speculate that the best cross-protection can be achieved only with the most stable and conserved particle structures. Additional Lassa antigens, such as NP or Z, which provide conserved epitopes as well as increase the formation of stable ribonucleoprotein particles, are predicted to increase vaccine breadth. A rigorous test of vaccine cross-protection or breadth must ultimately occur in primates.

Table 1. Comparison of select Lassa vaccine candidates.

Vaccine	Breadth of Cross-Protection [a]	Safety for Pregnant Women and Fetus [b]	Sterilizing Immunity [c]	Production Costs [d]	References
ML29 [e]	High	Low	Yes	Low	[16]
$MOPVAC_{LasGP}$ [f]	ND [g]	Low	Yes	Med	[86]
VSV-LAS_{GP} [h]	Med	Low	No	Med	[81]
MVA-LAS_{GP+Z} [i]	ND	High	ND	Med	[87]
$LASV_{GPC}$ DNA [j]	ND	High	Yes	High	[88]

[a] Refers to protection from distantly-related virus isolates. [b] This is a guess based on the propensity of similar viruses to cause fetal malformations or miscarriage. [c] Sterilizing immunity means that, after immunizing with an effective dose, there is no trace of the vaccine a week after immunization, neither in tissue nor in excreta. [d] Production costs are extrapolated from reported doses and levels of virus (or RNA) production in cell culture. [e] Mopeia/Lassa reassortant 29 (ML29) has the L RNA of Mopeia and the S RNA of $Lassa_{Josiah}$. It was selected from a library of MOPV/LASV reassortants for small-plaque phenotype, attenuation in mice, genotype from MOPV L RNA and LASV S RNA, genetic stability, and efficient replication in Vero cell cultures (~10^8 plaque forming units (pfu)/mL) [14]. The Russian laboratories of Fort, LLC have produced a variety of Mopeia/Lassa reassortants to improve upon the vaccine efficacy and patent protections of the initial isolates (Moshkoff D. and Nasidi A. in preparation). [f] MOPVAC or Mopeia-ExoNb6 (MOPV-ExoNb6) is a recombinant virus expressing the Mopeia genome, six mutations in the MOPV-NP exonuclease, and the LASV GP in place of the MOPV GP [86]. [g] ND means not determined. [h] VSV-LAS_{GP} refers to vaccines using the vesicular stomatitis virus (VSV) platform and expressing the Lassa GP. Both current versions have reduced neurovirulence: the Feldmann/Merck version has been attenuated by replacing the VSV G with the Lassa GP [89], and the Rose/Profectus version has been attenuated by altering the natural VSV gene order [90]. Both have reduced growth capacity compared to VSV, and, from our experience with other VSV pseudotypes, it is likely that they fail to reach titers above 10^7 plaque-forming units (pfu)/mL. [i] The GeoVax-made vaccine replicates well in avian cells but does not replicate in mammals. In mammals, it expresses LASV GP and Z genes, forming virus-like-particles (VLP) in vivo. The Modified Vaccinia Ankara (MVA) vector was developed by B. Moss at NIH and has been used in thousands of human beings in the form of an AIDS vaccine [91]. VLP can be powerful and broadly-protective immunogens. [j] $LASV_{GPC}$ DNA vaccine.

The laboratory of Silvain Baize has recently described a new vaccine ($MOPVAC_{LasGP}$) that is a Mopeia recombinant bearing a $Lassa_{Josiah}$ glycoprotein (GP). It has been genetically engineered to have six missense mutations in the exonuclease portion of its nucleocapsid protein (NP), a portion that is known to suppress the antiviral IFN response by cleavage of PRR-detecting RNA. This MOPVAC has not been tested for cross-protection, but it is seen as a platform for insertion of sequences for each of the Lassa lineages. Whereas the wild-type virus can reach high titers in culture, this attenuated version (MOPV-ExoN6b) reaches titers that are two logs lower [86], so it may not be vigorous enough for scaled production. In addition, it is possible that the altered exonuclease would allow vaccine persistence in vivo.

No live-attenuated RNA virus vaccines are recommended for administration to pregnant women because all replicating RNA viruses tested have been teratogenic for live births from an infected pregnant host. This is likely because viral replication requires host molecules that are also needed for fetal development [92]. Amongst the Lassa vaccines listed above, the first three are live-attenuated RNA viruses, whereas the last two, MVA and DNA vaccines, are not able to replicate in mammals, so are likely to be safe for pregnant human subjects.

All five listed vaccines can be altered by reverse genetics. A recombinant ML29 (rML29) has recently been rescued from cDNA clones. Using rML29 and tri-segmented technology, additional genes of interest (eGFP, Ebola GP, and *Plasmodium berghei* antigens) have been expressed in rML29 [93]. Thus, rML29 can be used as a potent vaccine platform for expressing arenaviral genes (e.g., LASV GP_{Pinneo} from distantly-related lineage I) and non-related antigens and immunomodulators.

At this time, only two Lassa vaccine candidates (ML29 and $VSV\text{-}Las_{GP}$) have demonstrated breadth of protection in guinea pigs; and only one, ML29, has shown the ability to protect against challenges from virus outside the lineage IV of $Lassa_{Josiah}$. After a head-to-head comparison, the ML29 and $VSV\text{-}Las_{GP}$ candidates should move forward in clinical trials targeting health care workers and other people on the front lines of an outbreak. The two vaccine candidates that do not replicate in mammals, MVA-LAS and LASV-DNA, and would consequently be more expensive to produce, should be reserved for clinical trials with children and pregnant women.

6. Improving the Humoral Immune Response to Lassa Vaccines

The humoral immune response appears late after infection and after experimental vaccination. HIV, LCMV, and Lassa viruses evade antibodies by mimicking self-glycoproteins and cloaking their foreign envelope glycoproteins with self-glycans [94–97]. The development of B cell responses to glycan-cloaked epitopes is a slow process that ultimately depends upon antigen density and the avidity of the antigens for the B cell receptors (BCR). Self-reactivity can be removed from antibodies by V(D)J recombination or hypermutation. For example, binding studies showed that only three mutations in a BCR could confer 50-fold lower binding to self-versus foreign antigens [98]. Helper T cells cooperate with anergic B cells only when BCR cross-linking by foreign antigen is greater than that induced by self-antigen [99]. The higher threshold to activate anergic B cells and recruit them to germinal centers can only be overcome by high antigen density or high affinity for the BCR. This means that low density GP on virions will fail to activate anergic B cells, especially if they have only moderate affinity for self-glycans. Consequently, the B cell arm of the antiviral immune response will only develop after exposure to high-density, high-affinity antigen.

Despite an initial cloaking of B cell antigens during viral infection, survivors acquire memory responses that increase over time. A study of 45 people who survived avian influenza showed that the sickest individuals, presumably those with highest viral titers, were the slowest to develop cell-mediated and humoral responses, but then they also developed the most long-term protective antibody responses [100].

The effort to make "universal flu vaccines" illustrates some approaches that could be used in making broadly-protective antibodies for Lassa virus disease. Initially, influenza researchers tried to increase the vaccine breadth by choosing immunogens such as the influenza hemagglutinin

(HA) stem that are most evolutionarily conserved. By choosing conserved antigens, one could vaccinate against the most stable portions of a pathogen and also achieve the greatest cross-protective immune responses. In one particular effort, a broadly-reactive vaccine was created by engineering a consensus of 2656 HA_{H1N1} protein sequences into one protein, CH1, that bore conserved B and T cell epitopes. A PR8-CH1 influenza virus elicited broadly-protective immunity against heterologous H1N1 viruses [101]. Researchers also considered using the neuraminidase (NA) since it is a less rapidly-evolving protein and thus a good contributor for vaccine antigens. Similarly, for arenaviruses such as LASV, the GP1 is highly variable, but a segment of GP2 and the NP are not very variable and therefore good antigens to include as immunogens.

It was recognized in the 1990s that the three-dimensional structure of an antigen contributed to the B cell response [102]. The contribution of large repetitive structures and conformational antigens to broadening the antigen response is an important approach that has been pursued in the search for universal influenza vaccines. Particulation of an antigen (e.g., putting it on a nanoparticle) leads to significant enhancement of BCR cross-linking and B cell activation [103]. B cell activation also leads to more activated CD4+ T cell responses, and promotion of antigen cross-presentation for CD8+ T cell activation [104]. Particulate antigens tend to cause auto-immunity, they are more frequently taken up by phagocytosis, they are DC-tropic, they are more immunogenic than soluble antigens, and they activate the inflammasome [105]. In agreement with these observations about particulation, vaccines comprised of virus particles or virus-like particles would be predicted to be more immunogenic than DNA vaccines or unstructured assemblages of viral antigens.

The production of VLP also exploits the particulation approach. The MVA-VLP vaccine results in highly structured antigens, in this case the Lassa Z (or matrix protein) in combination with the Lassa GP form VLP in vivo [87]. Stable particle formation for retroviruses also depends on two types of proteins: the envelope (Env) is thought to bear the most variable "type-specific antigens" while the abundant capsid protein "Gag" bears the more evolutionarily-stable "group-specific antigens" [106]. By adding Gag to a vaccine some investigators have been able to introduce evolutionarily-conserved regions that also contribute to a more stable ribonucleoprotein (RNP) structure [107].

The most conserved antigenic regions tend to include many non-linear (conformational) antigens that remain functionally stable during virus evolution. This finding is strengthened by the observation that roughly 60% of the neutralizing antibodies derived from convalescent Lassa patients relied on conformational epitopes [108]. A remarkable effort to characterize nAbs from convalescent human blood revealed that as antibodies matured over time, some antibodies were capable of neutralizing Lassa isolates from all four lineages, and some could neutralize LCMV as well as Lassa [108]. Unfortunately, it is well known that pseudotypes are more sensitive to nAbs than wild-type viruses [109,110], so this conclusion needs corroboration with LASV isolates. In these cases of broadly-neutralizing antibodies, breadth of neutralizing activity was dependent on conformational epitopes. It is a common theme that broadly-neutralizing anti-microbial antibodies bind to conformational epitopes, for example one of the broadest and most potent HIV neutralizing antibodies binds to the gp41–gp120 interface [111].

Leon et al., [112] showed that binding of large structured antigen-antibody complexes to Fc gamma receptor (FcγR) leads to stronger and more broadly cross-reactive B cell responses than antigens that elicit FcγR-independent antibodies. Antibodies that were hemaglutination (HA)-inhibiting tended to be FcγR-independent and antibodies that bound the conserved HA stalk structure tended to be FcγR-dependent. There was a large discrepancy between in vitro and in vivo assays for nAb efficacy: in vitro, HA stalk antibodies were 100–1000 fold weaker than HA-inhibiting antibodies, but in vivo passive transfer studies showed only a five-fold discrepancy between antibody efficacies. By testing a number of HA variants, this group found that the optimal nAb response requires, not only an interaction with FcγR, but also a second molecular bridge between pathogen and innate effector cells, serving perhaps to activate those cells. Antibodies against the influenza HA are more broadly reactive if they simultaneously engage both the FcγR and other pathogen-specific receptors on innate immune cells [112]. To translate this finding to enhancing the breadth of Lassa vaccines, those vaccines that engage both viral entry receptors and FcγR on innate immune cells should be the most broadly cross-protective immunogens. For example, a recent publication illustrates how a beta-propriolactone-inactivated Lassa-Rabies vector elicits lasting humoral responses against LASV and Rabies in mice and guinea pigs [113].

7. Improving the Cell-Mediated Immune Response to Lassa Infection

Memory T cells play a critical role in long-term protection against Lassa fever [74]. Nevertheless, the CD8+ T cell receptor (TCR) interaction with MHC-presented peptides is very constrained. 9mer epitopes in the context of MHC-class I must have a very tight and specific fit to the TCR to activate cytokine secretion or CTL activity. One strategy known as the "string of beads" approach was meant to increase vaccine breadth by including many of the primary epitopes in one expression vector. This was tried for AIDS and for arenavirus vaccines, but it resulted in a competition between similar epitopes so that the immune response became quickly focused but not broader [114]. A slightly different approach, stringing the non-dominant epitopes, succeeded in avoiding focus and developed a broader protective vaccine response [115]. Using adenoviral vectors expressing invariant chain-linked non-dominant LCMV GP antigen, the AR Thomsen and JP Christensen laboratories were able to show that efficient virus control may be obtained by targeting the intrinsically non-dominant GP antigen, and that this allows for a potent CD8 T cell response to be elicited by virus-encoded dominant NP antigen during the chronic phase of a high-dose infection. In contrast, when mice were initially vaccinated using the dominant NP antigen, the subsequent virus-elicited response remained focused on the major NP epitope. During the early period after virus challenge, it was possible to confirm that T cells primed by the Adeno-GP vaccine and boosted by the virus infection were able to protect against a broad array of challenge viruses [115].

Whereas class I peptides present to CD8 T cells and are constrained in size to anchor within the peptide groove of MHC class I molecules, class II peptides present to CD4 T cells and are much less constrained, varying from 11 to 30 amino acids in length [116]. An approach suggested by Dr. M. Patarroyo for synthetic-vaccine development is to determine immune protection-inducing protein structures (IMPIPS) by stringing together class II peptides. This involves defining the three-dimensional interactions which are essential in $MHC_{ClassII}$–peptide–Tcell receptor (TCR) complex formation, a much more promiscuous coupling activity than the interactions of class I peptides and CD8 TCR. After finding an orientation for perfectly fitting into the TCR that induces an appropriate immune response, non-interfering, long-lasting, protective, multi-epitope peptides can be synthesized against many infections [117,118]. Even non-immunogenic epitopes can be converted into immunogens using the Patarroyo TCR-binding selections, thereby avoiding the over-reaction problems caused by pre-existing immunity against microorganisms.

In AIDS vaccine research, there has also been an approach favoring class II epitopes. This is promising because it is well known that CD4+ TCR can be more frequently cross-restrictive than the CD8 TCR [116]. The ability to cross-restrict allowed AIDS Elite Controllers to have both avid TCR interactions with Gag293 epitope in the context of HLA-DR (class II) and to have broad cross-restriction between Gag and Env V2 epitopes. Thus, a broad cross-reactivity of CD4+ T cell responses, similar to that commonly seen in Elite Controllers, could be established by vaccination in ordinary individuals [119]. With respect to Lassa vaccines, it is likely that Lassa disease survivors bear some similarities to AIDS Elite Controllers in their acquired immunity, showing broadly cross-restricted CD4 responses. An understanding of the CD4 TCR alleles determining this response should make it possible to engineer autologous T cells that confer protection.

With high HLA heterogeneity among the West African population, the feasibility of epitope-based vaccines is limited. A safety issue was raised in murine experiments where epitope-based vaccines given to individuals who had previously been exposed to the pathogen can strongly re-activate the pre-existing CD8+ T clones and induce TNF-dependent immunopathology [120], but then this may be a murine problem and not a serious problem for human subjects.

8. Future Directions Combining Immunological and Drug-Therapy Approaches

When health care professionals are getting ready to risk their lives during an epidemic, a strong, fast-acting and broadly-protective vaccine should be available. The poor conditions and shear volume of needy patients makes a dangerous situation for first-responders and they deserve to be armed with protection. In addition to vaccines, broadly-protective antiviral therapies should be available. Both the ML29 and VSV-LAS vaccines have shown antiviral efficacy when used within two days of Lassa infection [16,81], however their action within this brief window of time is lineage-specific rather than broadly protective. It is telling that a repatriated health care worker who ultimately survived was given intravenous fluids and two broadly acting antivirals (ribavirin pn days 6–15 of illness and favipiravir days 8–12 of illness) [74]. Nevertheless, it is still unclear whether the optimum care requires anything more than intravenous fluids and good hospital practices.

Several studies have yielded broadly cross-protective antivirals that could be used against Lassa infection. High-throughput screens for small molecule inhibitors of LASV revealed an inhibitor of arenavirus polymerases (favipiravir) that was recently used on a LASV-infected health care worker along with intravenous fluids and ribavirin [74]. This treatment is so broadly cross-protective it has even been used on Ebola cases [121]. Ribavirin also has broad reactivity against many RNA viruses and at its lowest concentration works by blocking the capped-mRNA-promoting function of eIF4E [122]. Unfortunately, ribavirin resistance is problematic; thus, it is best used in combination with other antivirals [123]. A recent study of the interactome of LCMV gene products with host cell molecules revealed several host-cell molecules essential to the life cycle of viruses including Junin, LASV and Ebola [124,125]. Mining such data will yield a steady pipeline of antiviral approaches that could protect simultaneously against several viruses. The standard of care for patients may eventually include both rapid-acting vaccines and broadly-acting antiviral drugs.

In summary, there is an urgent need for head-to-head comparisons of the current popular vaccine candidates because their relative stabilities, production capacities, and protective breadth in primates remain unknown. Having established such a comparison, two types of vaccines should be developed: a cheaply-produced vaccine (e.g., ML29 or VSV-LAS) for emergency use in endemic areas, and a more expensive vaccine (e.g. the MVA or DNA vaccines) for vulnerable populations such as pregnant women. These two types of vaccines can be further improved by increasing immunity to conformational antigens or by favoring epitopes known to bind tightly to HLA and cross-restrict with conformational antigens. After following this path to improving the current popular Lassa vaccine candidates, treatments combining vaccines and therapeutic drugs should be optimized as well.

Author Contributions: J.C.Z., S.M.-M., C.G.-C. and M.S.S. reviewed the literature and wrote the manuscript.

Funding: This research was funded by NIH/NIAID-supported awards: R01 AI052367 and R01 AI068961 to IS Lukashevich, and 5RC2CA149001 from NCI and R21-AI074790 to MS Salvato. Support also came from the EU Commission Horizon2020 STARBIOS2 grant No. 709517 under Vittorio Colizzi in accord with five key tenets of Responsible Research and Innovation: Public Engagement, Gender Equity, Open Access, Graduate Education, and Ethical conduct.

Acknowledgments: We like to thank I.S. Lukashevich for providing critical remarks and comments.

Conflicts of Interest: The authors declare no conflict of interest.

References

1. Fichet-Calvet, E.; Rogers, D.J. Risk maps of lassa fever in west africa. *PLoS Negl Trop Dis* **2009**, *3*, e388. [CrossRef] [PubMed]
2. WHO. Ebola Situation Report-17. 2016. Available online: http://apps.who.int/ebola/ebola-situation-reports (accessed on 20 October 2018).

3. CEPI. Coalition for Epidemic Preparedness Innovations (Cepi) Inception and Top Bio-Threats. 2017. Available online: http://www.who.int/medicines/ebola-treatment/TheCoalitionEpidemicPreparednessInnovations-an-overview.pdf (accessed on 20 October 2018).
4. WHO. Lassa Roadmap Meeting. 2018. Available online: http://www.who.int/blueprint/priority-diseases/key-action/lassa-fever/en/ (accessed on 20 October 2018).
5. Bowen, M.D.; Rollin, P.E.; Ksiazek, T.G.; Hustad, H.L.; Bausch, D.G.; Demby, A.H.; Bajani, M.D.; Peters, C.J.; Nichol, S.T. Genetic diversity among lassa virus strains. *J. Virol.* **2000**, *74*, 6992–7004. [CrossRef] [PubMed]
6. Andersen, K.G.; Shapiro, B.J.; Matranga, C.B.; Sealfon, R.; Lin, A.E.; Moses, L.M.; Folarin, O.A.; Goba, A.; Odia, I.; Ehiane, P.E.; et al. Clinical sequencing uncovers origins and evolution of lassa virus. *Cell* **2015**, *162*, 738–750. [CrossRef] [PubMed]
7. Siddle, K.J.; Eromon, P.; Barnes, K.G.; Mehta, S.; Oguzie, J.U.; Odia, I.; Schaffner, S.F.; Winnicki, S.M.; Shah, R.R.; Qu, J.; et al. Genomic analysis of lassa virus during an increase in cases in nigeria in 2018. *N. Engl. J. Med.* **2018**. [CrossRef] [PubMed]
8. Weidmann, M.; Sall, A.A.; Manuguerra, J.C.; Koivogui, L.; Adjami, A.; Traore, F.F.; Hedlund, K.O.; Lindegren, G.; Mirazimi, A. Quantitative analysis of particles, genomes and infectious particles in supernatants of haemorrhagic fever virus cell cultures. *Virol. J.* **2011**, *8*, 81. [CrossRef] [PubMed]
9. Emonet, S.; Lemasson, J.J.; Gonzalez, J.P.; de Lamballerie, X.; Charrel, R.N. Phylogeny and evolution of old world arenaviruses. *Virology* **2006**, *350*, 251–257. [CrossRef] [PubMed]
10. Lukashevich, I.S.; Maryankova, R.; Vladyko, A.S.; Nashkevich, N.; Koleda, S.; Djavani, M.; Horejsh, D.; Voitenok, N.N.; Salvato, M.S. Lassa and mopeia virus replication in human monocytes/macrophages and in endothelial cells: Different effects on il-8 and tnf-alpha gene expression. *J. Med. Virol.* **1999**, *59*, 552–560. [CrossRef]
11. Baize, S.; Kaplon, J.; Faure, C.; Pannetier, D.; Georges-Courbot, M.C.; Deubel, V. Lassa virus infection of human dendritic cells and macrophages is productive but fails to activate cells. *J. Immunol.* **2004**, *172*, 2861–2869. [CrossRef] [PubMed]
12. Pannetier, D.; Reynard, S.; Russier, M.; Journeaux, A.; Tordo, N.; Deubel, V.; Baize, S. Human dendritic cells infected with the nonpathogenic mopeia virus induce stronger t-cell responses than those infected with lassa virus. *J. Virol.* **2011**, *85*, 8293–8306. [CrossRef] [PubMed]
13. Sommerstein, R.; Flatz, L.; Remy, M.M.; Malinge, P.; Magistrelli, G.; Fischer, N.; Sahin, M.; Bergthaler, A.; Igonet, S.; Ter Meulen, J.; et al. Arenavirus glycan shield promotes neutralizing antibody evasion and protracted infection. *PLoS Pathog.* **2015**, *11*, e1005276. [CrossRef] [PubMed]
14. Lukashevich, I.S. Generation of reassortants between african arenaviruses. *Virology* **1992**, *188*, 600–605. [CrossRef]
15. Lukashevich, I.S.; Patterson, J.; Carrion, R.; Moshkoff, D.; Ticer, A.; Zapata, J.; Brasky, K.; Geiger, R.; Hubbard, G.B.; Bryant, J.; et al. A live attenuated vaccine for lassa fever made by reassortment of lassa and mopeia viruses. *J. Virol.* **2005**, *79*, 13934–13942. [CrossRef] [PubMed]
16. Carrion, R., Jr.; Patterson, J.L.; Johnson, C.; Gonzales, M.; Moreira, C.R.; Ticer, A.; Brasky, K.; Hubbard, G.B.; Moshkoff, D.; Zapata, J.; et al. A ml29 reassortant virus protects guinea pigs against a distantly related nigerian strain of lassa virus and can provide sterilizing immunity. *Vaccine* **2007**, *25*, 4093–4102. [CrossRef] [PubMed]
17. Moshkoff, D.A.; Salvato, M.S.; Lukashevich, I.S. Molecular characterization of a reassortant virus derived from lassa and mopeia viruses. *Virus Genes* **2007**, *34*, 169–176. [CrossRef] [PubMed]
18. Lukashevich, I.S.; Carrion, R., Jr.; Salvato, M.S.; Mansfield, K.; Brasky, K.; Zapata, J.; Cairo, C.; Goicochea, M.; Hoosien, G.E.; Ticer, A.; et al. Safety, immunogenicity, and efficacy of the ml29 reassortant vaccine for lassa fever in small non-human primates. *Vaccine* **2008**, *26*, 5246–5254. [CrossRef] [PubMed]
19. Zapata, J.C.; Poonia, B.; Bryant, J.; Davis, H.; Ateh, E.; George, L.; Crasta, O.; Zhang, Y.; Slezak, T.; Jaing, C.; et al. An attenuated lassa vaccine in siv-infected rhesus macaques does not persist or cause arenavirus disease but does elicit lassa virus-specific immunity. *Virol. J.* **2013**, *10*, 52. [CrossRef] [PubMed]
20. Johnson, K.M.; McCormick, J.B.; Webb, P.A.; Smith, E.S.; Elliott, L.H.; King, I.J. Clinical virology of lassa fever in hospitalized patients. *J. Infect. Dis.* **1987**, *155*, 456–464. [CrossRef] [PubMed]
21. Oldstone, M.B.; Campbell, K.P. Decoding arenavirus pathogenesis: Essential roles for alpha-dystroglycan-virus interactions and the immune response. *Virology* **2011**, *411*, 170–179. [CrossRef] [PubMed]

22. Schmitz, H.; Kohler, B.; Laue, T.; Drosten, C.; Veldkamp, P.J.; Gunther, S.; Emmerich, P.; Geisen, H.P.; Fleischer, K.; Beersma, M.F.; et al. Monitoring of clinical and laboratory data in two cases of imported lassa fever. *Microbes Infect.* **2002**, *4*, 43–50. [CrossRef]
23. Jahrling, P.B.; Frame, J.D.; Rhoderick, J.B.; Monson, M.H. Endemic lassa fever in liberia. Iv. Selection of optimally effective plasma for treatment by passive immunization. *Trans. R. Soc. Trop. Med. Hyg.* **1985**, *79*, 380–384. [CrossRef]
24. McCormick, J.B.; Walker, D.H.; King, I.J.; Webb, P.A.; Elliott, L.H.; Whitfield, S.G.; Johnson, K.M. Lassa virus hepatitis: A study of fatal lassa fever in humans. *Am. J. Trop. Med. Hyg.* **1986**, *35*, 401–407. [CrossRef] [PubMed]
25. Carrion, R., Jr.; Brasky, K.; Mansfield, K.; Johnson, C.; Gonzales, M.; Ticer, A.; Lukashevich, I.; Tardif, S.; Patterson, J. Lassa virus infection in experimentally infected marmosets: Liver pathology and immunophenotypic alterations in target tissues. *J. Virol.* **2007**, *81*, 6482–6490. [CrossRef] [PubMed]
26. Fedeli, C.; Torriani, G.; Galan-Navarro, C.; Moraz, M.L.; Moreno, H.; Gerold, G.; Kunz, S. Axl can serve as entry factor for lassa virus depending on the functional glycosylation of dystroglycan. *J. Virol.* **2018**, *92*, e01613-17. [CrossRef] [PubMed]
27. Beier, J.I.; Jokinen, J.D.; Holz, G.E.; Whang, P.S.; Martin, A.M.; Warner, N.L.; Arteel, G.E.; Lukashevich, I.S. Novel mechanism of arenavirus-induced liver pathology. *PLoS ONE* **2015**, *10*, e0122839. [CrossRef] [PubMed]
28. Cummins, D.; Fisher-Hoch, S.P.; Walshe, K.J.; Mackie, I.J.; McCormick, J.B.; Bennett, D.; Perez, G.; Farrar, B.; Machin, S.J. A plasma inhibitor of platelet aggregation in patients with lassa fever. *Br. J. Haematol.* **1989**, *72*, 543–548. [CrossRef] [PubMed]
29. Fisher-Hoch, S.; McCormick, J.B.; Sasso, D.; Craven, R.B. Hematologic dysfunction in lassa fever. *J. Med. Virol.* **1988**, *26*, 127–135. [CrossRef] [PubMed]
30. Fisher-Hoch, S.P.; McCormick, J.B. Pathophysiology and treatment of lassa fever. *Curr. Top. Microbiol. Immunol.* **1987**, *134*, 231–239. [PubMed]
31. Knobloch, J.; McCormick, J.B.; Webb, P.A.; Dietrich, M.; Schumacher, H.H.; Dennis, E. Clinical observations in 42 patients with lassa fever. *Tropenmed. Parasitol.* **1980**, *31*, 389–398. [PubMed]
32. Lange, J.V.; Mitchell, S.W.; McCormick, J.B.; Walker, D.H.; Evatt, B.L.; Ramsey, R.R. Kinetic study of platelets and fibrinogen in lassa virus-infected monkeys and early pathologic events in mopeia virus-infected monkeys. *Am. J. Trop. Med. Hyg.* **1985**, *34*, 999–1007. [CrossRef] [PubMed]
33. Cummins, D.; McCormick, J.B.; Bennett, D.; Samba, J.A.; Farrar, B.; Machin, S.J.; Fisher-Hoch, S.P. Acute sensorineural deafness in lassa fever. *JAMA* **1990**, *264*, 2093–2096. [CrossRef] [PubMed]
34. Fisher-Hoch, S.P.; Mitchell, S.W.; Sasso, D.R.; Lange, J.V.; Ramsey, R.; McCormick, J.B. Physiological and immunologic disturbances associated with shock in a primate model of lassa fever. *J. Infect. Dis.* **1987**, *155*, 465–474. [CrossRef] [PubMed]
35. Khan, S.H.; Goba, A.; Chu, M.; Roth, C.; Healing, T.; Marx, A.; Fair, J.; Guttieri, M.C.; Ferro, P.; Imes, T.; et al. New opportunities for field research on the pathogenesis and treatment of lassa fever. *Antivir. Res.* **2008**, *78*, 103–115. [CrossRef] [PubMed]
36. Peters, C.J.; Liu, C.T.; Anderson, G.W., Jr.; Morrill, J.C.; Jahrling, P.B. Pathogenesis of viral hemorrhagic fevers: Rift valley fever and lassa fever contrasted. *Rev. Infect. Dis.* **1989**, *11* (Suppl. 4), S743–S749. [CrossRef]
37. Solbrig, M.V. Headache syndromes in sierra leone, west africa. *Headache* **1991**, *31*, 419. [PubMed]
38. Baize, S.; Marianneau, P.; Loth, P.; Reynard, S.; Journeaux, A.; Chevallier, M.; Tordo, N.; Deubel, V.; Contamin, H. Early and strong immune responses are associated with control of viral replication and recovery in lassa virus-infected cynomolgus monkeys. *J. Virol.* **2009**, *83*, 5890–5903. [CrossRef] [PubMed]
39. Edington, G.M.; White, H.A. The pathology of lassa fever. *Trans. R. Soc. Trop. Med. Hyg.* **1972**, *66*, 381–389. [CrossRef]
40. Hensley, L.E.; Smith, M.A.; Geisbert, J.B.; Fritz, E.A.; Daddario-DiCaprio, K.M.; Larsen, T.; Geisbert, T.W. Pathogenesis of lassa fever in cynomolgus macaques. *Virol. J.* **2011**, *8*, 205. [CrossRef] [PubMed]
41. McCormick, J.B.; Fisher-Hoch, S.P. Lassa fever. *Curr. Top. Microbiol. Immunol.* **2002**, *262*, 75–109. [PubMed]
42. Mahanty, S.; Hutchinson, K.; Agarwal, S.; McRae, M.; Rollin, P.E.; Pulendran, B. Cutting edge: Impairment of dendritic cells and adaptive immunity by ebola and lassa viruses. *J. Immunol.* **2003**, *170*, 2797–2801. [CrossRef] [PubMed]
43. Jacobs, B.L.; Langland, J.O. When two strands are better than one: The mediators and modulators of the cellular responses to double-stranded rna. *Virology* **1996**, *219*, 339–349. [CrossRef] [PubMed]

44. Kell, A.M.; Gale, M., Jr. Rig-i in rna virus recognition. *Virology* **2015**, *479–480*, 110–121. [CrossRef] [PubMed]
45. Asper, M.; Sternsdorf, T.; Hass, M.; Drosten, C.; Rhode, A.; Schmitz, H.; Gunther, S. Inhibition of different lassa virus strains by alpha and gamma interferons and comparison with a less pathogenic arenavirus. *J. Virol.* **2004**, *78*, 3162–3169. [CrossRef] [PubMed]
46. Lukashevich, I.S.; Tikhonov, I.; Rodas, J.D.; Zapata, J.C.; Yang, Y.; Djavani, M.; Salvato, M.S. Arenavirus-mediated liver pathology: Acute lymphocytic choriomeningitis virus infection of rhesus macaques is characterized by high-level interleukin-6 expression and hepatocyte proliferation. *J. Virol.* **2003**, *77*, 1727–1737. [CrossRef] [PubMed]
47. Branco, L.M.; Grove, J.N.; Boisen, M.L.; Shaffer, J.G.; Goba, A.; Fullah, M.; Momoh, M.; Grant, D.S.; Garry, R.F. Emerging trends in lassa fever: Redefining the role of immunoglobulin m and inflammation in diagnosing acute infection. *Virol. J.* **2011**, *8*, 478. [CrossRef] [PubMed]
48. Martinez-Sobrido, L.; Emonet, S.; Giannakas, P.; Cubitt, B.; Garcia-Sastre, A.; de la Torre, J.C. Identification of amino acid residues critical for the anti-interferon activity of the nucleoprotein of the prototypic arenavirus lymphocytic choriomeningitis virus. *J. Virol.* **2009**, *83*, 11330–11340. [CrossRef] [PubMed]
49. Hastie, K.M.; Kimberlin, C.R.; Zandonatti, M.A.; MacRae, I.J.; Saphire, E.O. Structure of the lassa virus nucleoprotein reveals a dsrna-specific 3′ to 5′ exonuclease activity essential for immune suppression. *Proc. Natl. Acad. Sci. USA* **2011**, *108*, 2396–2401. [CrossRef] [PubMed]
50. Martinez-Sobrido, L.; Giannakas, P.; Cubitt, B.; Garcia-Sastre, A.; de la Torre, J.C. Differential inhibition of type i interferon induction by arenavirus nucleoproteins. *J. Virol.* **2007**, *81*, 12696–12703. [CrossRef] [PubMed]
51. Martinez-Sobrido, L.; Zuniga, E.I.; Rosario, D.; Garcia-Sastre, A.; de la Torre, J.C. Inhibition of the type i interferon response by the nucleoprotein of the prototypic arenavirus lymphocytic choriomeningitis virus. *J. Virol.* **2006**, *80*, 9192–9199. [CrossRef] [PubMed]
52. Qi, X.; Lan, S.; Wang, W.; Schelde, L.M.; Dong, H.; Wallat, G.D.; Ly, H.; Liang, Y.; Dong, C. Cap binding and immune evasion revealed by lassa nucleoprotein structure. *Nature* **2010**, *468*, 779–783. [CrossRef] [PubMed]
53. Zhou, S.; Cerny, A.M.; Zacharia, A.; Fitzgerald, K.A.; Kurt-Jones, E.A.; Finberg, R.W. Induction and inhibition of type i interferon responses by distinct components of lymphocytic choriomeningitis virus. *J. Virol.* **2010**, *84*, 9452–9462. [CrossRef] [PubMed]
54. Xing, J.; Ly, H.; Liang, Y. The z proteins of pathogenic but not nonpathogenic arenaviruses inhibit rig-i-like receptor-dependent interferon production. *J. Virol.* **2015**, *89*, 2944–2955. [CrossRef] [PubMed]
55. Forni, D.; Pontremoli, C.; Pozzoli, U.; Clerici, M.; Cagliani, R.; Sironi, M. Ancient evolution of mammarenaviruses: Adaptation via changes in the l protein and no evidence for host-virus codivergence. *Genome Biol. Evol.* **2018**, *10*, 863–874. [CrossRef] [PubMed]
56. Grove, J.N.; Branco, L.M.; Boisen, M.L.; Muncy, I.J.; Henderson, L.A.; Schieffellin, J.S.; Robinson, J.E.; Bangura, J.J.; Fonnie, M.; Schoepp, R.J.; et al. Capacity building permitting comprehensive monitoring of a severe case of lassa hemorrhagic fever in sierra leone with a positive outcome: Case report. *Virol. J.* **2011**, *8*, 314. [CrossRef] [PubMed]
57. Djavani, M.M.; Crasta, O.R.; Zapata, J.C.; Fei, Z.; Folkerts, O.; Sobral, B.; Swindells, M.; Bryant, J.; Davis, H.; Pauza, C.D.; et al. Early blood profiles of virus infection in a monkey model for lassa fever. *J. Virol.* **2007**, *81*, 7960–7973. [CrossRef] [PubMed]
58. Hayes, M.W.; Carrion, R., Jr.; Nunneley, J.; Medvedev, A.E.; Salvato, M.S.; Lukashevich, I.S. Pathogenic old world arenaviruses inhibit tlr2/mal-dependent proinflammatory cytokines in vitro. *J. Virol.* **2012**, *86*, 7216–7226. [CrossRef] [PubMed]
59. Lukashevich, I.S.; Rodas, J.D.; Tikhonov, I.I.; Zapata, J.C.; Yang, Y.; Djavani, M.; Salvato, M.S. Lcmv-mediated hepatitis in rhesus macaques: We but not arm strain activates hepatocytes and induces liver regeneration. *Arch. Virol.* **2004**, *149*, 2319–2336. [CrossRef] [PubMed]
60. McCormick, J.B.; Mitchell, S.W.; Kiley, M.P.; Ruo, S.; Fisher-Hoch, S.P. Inactivated lassa virus elicits a non protective immune response in rhesus monkeys. *J. Med. Virol.* **1992**, *37*, 1–7. [CrossRef] [PubMed]
61. Arnold, R.B.; Gary, G.W. A neutralization test survey for lassa fever activity in lassa, nigeria. *Trans. R. Soc. Trop. Med. Hyg.* **1977**, *71*, 152–154. [CrossRef]
62. Lukashevich, I.S.; Clegg, J.C.; Sidibe, K. Lassa virus activity in guinea: Distribution of human antiviral antibody defined using enzyme-linked immunosorbent assay with recombinant antigen. *J. Med. Virol.* **1993**, *40*, 210–217. [CrossRef] [PubMed]

63. Tomori, O.; Fabiyi, A.; Sorungbe, A.; Smith, A.; McCormick, J.B. Viral hemorrhagic fever antibodies in nigerian populations. *Am. J. Trop. Med. Hyg.* **1988**, *38*, 407–410. [CrossRef] [PubMed]
64. McCormick, J.B.; Webb, P.A.; Krebs, J.W.; Johnson, K.M.; Smith, E.S. A prospective study of the epidemiology and ecology of lassa fever. *J. Infect. Dis.* **1987**, *155*, 437–444. [CrossRef] [PubMed]
65. Fisher-Hoch, S.P.; McCormick, J.B. Towards a human lassa fever vaccine. *Rev. Med. Virol.* **2001**, *11*, 331–341. [CrossRef] [PubMed]
66. Leifer, E.; Gocke, D.J.; Bourne, H. Lassa fever, a new virus disease of man from west africa. Ii. Report of a laboratory-acquired infection treated with plasma from a person recently recovered from the disease. *Am. J. Trop. Med. Hyg.* **1970**, *19*, 677–679. [CrossRef] [PubMed]
67. McCormick, J.B.; King, I.J.; Webb, P.A.; Scribner, C.L.; Craven, R.B.; Johnson, K.M.; Elliott, L.H.; Belmont-Williams, R. Lassa fever. Effective therapy with ribavirin. *N. Engl. J. Med.* **1986**, *314*, 20–26. [CrossRef] [PubMed]
68. Mire, C.E.; Cross, R.W.; Geisbert, J.B.; Borisevich, V.; Agans, K.N.; Deer, D.J.; Heinrich, M.L.; Rowland, M.M.; Goba, A.; Momoh, M.; et al. Human-monoclonal-antibody therapy protects nonhuman primates against advanced lassa fever. *Nat. Med.* **2017**, *23*, 1146–1149. [CrossRef] [PubMed]
69. Hastie, K.M.; Saphire, E.O. Lassa virus glycoprotein: Stopping a moving target. *Curr. Opin. Virol.* **2018**, *31*, 52–58. [CrossRef] [PubMed]
70. Fisher-Hoch, S.P.; McCormick, J.B. Lassa fever vaccine. *Expert Rev. Vaccines* **2004**, *3*, 189–197. [CrossRef] [PubMed]
71. Richmond, J.K.; Baglole, D.J. Lassa fever: Epidemiology, clinical features, and social consequences. *Br. Med. J.* **2003**, *327*, 1271–1275. [CrossRef] [PubMed]
72. ter Meulen, J.; Badusche, M.; Kuhnt, K.; Doetze, A.; Satoguina, J.; Marti, T.; Loeliger, C.; Koulemou, K.; Koivogui, L.; Schmitz, H.; et al. Characterization of human CD4(+) t-cell clones recognizing conserved and variable epitopes of the lassa virus nucleoprotein. *J. Virol.* **2000**, *74*, 2186–2192. [CrossRef] [PubMed]
73. Meulen, J.; Badusche, M.; Satoguina, J.; Strecker, T.; Lenz, O.; Loeliger, C.; Sakho, M.; Koulemou, K.; Koivogui, L.; Hoerauf, A. Old and new world arenaviruses share a highly conserved epitope in the fusion domain of the glycoprotein 2, which is recognized by lassa virus-specific human cd4+ t-cell clones. *Virology* **2004**, *321*, 134–143. [CrossRef] [PubMed]
74. McElroy, A.K.; Akondy, R.S.; Harmon, J.R.; Ellebedy, A.H.; Cannon, D.; Klena, J.D.; Sidney, J.; Sette, A.; Mehta, A.K.; Kraft, C.S.; et al. A case of human lassa virus infection with robust acute t-cell activation and long-term virus-specific t-cell responses. *J. Infect. Dis.* **2017**, *215*, 1862–1872. [CrossRef] [PubMed]
75. Goicochea, M.A.; Zapata, J.C.; Bryant, J.; Davis, H.; Salvato, M.S.; Lukashevich, I.S. Evaluation of lassa virus vaccine immunogenicity in a cba/j-ml29 mouse model. *Vaccine* **2012**, *30*, 1445–1452. [CrossRef] [PubMed]
76. Jahrling, P.B.; Peters, C.J. Serology and virulence diversity among old-world arenaviruses, and the relevance to vaccine development. *Med. Microbiol. Immunol.* **1986**, *175*, 165–167. [CrossRef] [PubMed]
77. Pushko, P.; Geisbert, J.; Parker, M.; Jahrling, P.; Smith, J. Individual and bivalent vaccines based on alphavirus replicons protect guinea pigs against infection with lassa and ebola viruses. *J. Virol.* **2001**, *75*, 11677–11685. [CrossRef] [PubMed]
78. Kiley, M.P.; Lange, J.V.; Johnson, K.M. Protection of rhesus monkeys from lassa virus by immunisation with closely related arenavirus. *Lancet* **1979**, *2*, 738. [CrossRef]
79. Walker, D.H.; Johnson, K.M.; Lange, J.V.; Gardner, J.J.; Kiley, M.P.; McCormick, J.B. Experimental infection of rhesus monkeys with lassa virus and a closely related arenavirus, mozambique virus. *J. Infect. Dis.* **1982**, *146*, 360–368. [CrossRef] [PubMed]
80. Maes, P.; Alkhovsky, S.V.; Bao, Y.; Beer, M.; Birkhead, M.; Briese, T.; Buchmeier, M.J.; Calisher, C.H.; Charrel, R.N.; Choi, I.R.; et al. Taxonomy of the family arenaviridae and the order bunyavirales: Update 2018. *Arch. Virol.* **2018**, *163*, 2295–2310. [CrossRef] [PubMed]
81. Safronetz, D.; Mire, C.; Rosenke, K.; Feldmann, F.; Haddock, E.; Geisbert, T.; Feldmann, H. A recombinant vesicular stomatitis virus-based lassa fever vaccine protects guinea pigs and macaques against challenge with geographically and genetically distinct lassa viruses. *PLoS Negl. Trop. Dis.* **2015**, *9*, e0003736. [CrossRef] [PubMed]
82. Clegg, J.C.; Lloyd, G. Vaccinia recombinant expressing lassa-virus internal nucleocapsid protein protects guineapigs against lassa fever. *Lancet* **1987**, *2*, 186–188. [CrossRef]

83. Peters, C.J.; Jahrling, P.B.; Liu, C.T.; Kenyon, R.H.; McKee, K.T., Jr.; Barrera Oro, J.G. Experimental studies of arenaviral hemorrhagic fevers. *Curr. Top. Microbiol. Immunol.* **1987**, *134*, 5–68. [PubMed]
84. Bredenbeek, P.J.; Molenkamp, R.; Spaan, W.J.; Deubel, V.; Marianneau, P.; Salvato, M.S.; Moshkoff, D.; Zapata, J.; Tikhonov, I.; Patterson, J.; et al. A recombinant yellow fever 17d vaccine expressing lassa virus glycoproteins. *Virology* **2006**, *345*, 299–304. [CrossRef] [PubMed]
85. Jiang, X.; Dalebout, T.J.; Bredenbeek, P.J.; Carrion, R., Jr.; Brasky, K.; Patterson, J.; Goicochea, M.; Bryant, J.; Salvato, M.S.; Lukashevich, I.S. Yellow fever 17d-vectored vaccines expressing lassa virus gp1 and gp2 glycoproteins provide protection against fatal disease in guinea pigs. *Vaccine* **2011**, *29*, 1248–1257. [CrossRef] [PubMed]
86. Carnec, X.; Mateo, M.; Page, A.; Reynard, S.; Hortion, J.; Picard, C.; Yekwa, E.; Barrot, L.; Barron, S.; Vallve, A.; et al. A vaccine platform against arenaviruses based on a recombinant hyperattenuated mopeia virus expressing heterologous glycoproteins. *J. Virol.* **2018**, *92*, e02230-17. [CrossRef] [PubMed]
87. Salvato, M.S.; Domi, A.; Guzmán-Cardozo, C.; Zapata, J.C.; Medina-Moreno, S.; Hsu, H.; McCurley, N.P.; Basu, R.; Hauser, M.; Hellerstein, M.S.; et al. A single dose of modified vaccinia ankara expressing lassa virus like particles protects mice from lethal intracerebral virus challenge. *Sci. Rep.* **2018**, in preparation.
88. Cashman, K.A.; Wilkinson, E.R.; Shaia, C.I.; Facemire, P.R.; Bell, T.M.; Bearss, J.J.; Shamblin, J.D.; Wollen, S.E.; Broderick, K.E.; Sardesai, N.Y.; et al. A DNA vaccine delivered by dermal electroporation fully protects cynomolgus macaques against lassa fever. *Hum. Vaccin. Immunother.* **2017**, *13*, 2902–2911. [CrossRef] [PubMed]
89. Geisbert, T.W.; Jones, S.; Fritz, E.A.; Shurtleff, A.C.; Geisbert, J.B.; Liebscher, R.; Grolla, A.; Stroher, U.; Fernando, L.; Daddario, K.M.; et al. Development of a new vaccine for the prevention of lassa fever. *PLoS Med.* **2005**, *2*, e183. [CrossRef] [PubMed]
90. Clarke, D.K.; Hendry, R.M.; Singh, V.; Rose, J.K.; Seligman, S.J.; Klug, B.; Kochhar, S.; Mac, L.M.; Carbery, B.; Chen, R.T.; et al. Live virus vaccines based on a vesicular stomatitis virus (vsv) backbone: Standardized template with key considerations for a risk/benefit assessment. *Vaccine* **2016**, *34*, 6597–6609. [CrossRef] [PubMed]
91. Kim, J.H.; Excler, J.L.; Michael, N.L. Lessons from the rv144 thai phase iii hiv-1 vaccine trial and the search for correlates of protection. *Annu. Rev. Med.* **2015**, *66*, 423–437. [CrossRef] [PubMed]
92. Djavani, M.; Topisirovic, I.; Zapata, J.C.; Sadowska, M.; Yang, Y.; Rodas, J.; Lukashevich, I.S.; Bogue, C.W.; Pauza, C.D.; Borden, K.L.; et al. The proline-rich homeodomain (prh/hex) protein is down-regulated in liver during infection with lymphocytic choriomeningitis virus. *J. Virol.* **2005**, *79*, 2461–2473. [CrossRef] [PubMed]
93. Iwasaki, M.; Cubitt, B.; Jokinen, J.; Lukashevich, I.S.; de la Torre, J.C. Use of recombinant ml29 platform to generate polyvalent live-attenuated vaccines against lassa fever and other infectious diseases. In Proceedings of the 66th Annual Meeting of Japanese Society for Virology, Kyoto, Japan, 28–30 October 2018.
94. Haynes, B.F.; Verkoczy, L. Aids/hiv. Host controls of hiv neutralizing antibodies. *Science* **2014**, *344*, 588–589. [CrossRef] [PubMed]
95. Pinschewer, D.D.; Perez, M.; Jeetendra, E.; Bachi, T.; Horvath, E.; Hengartner, H.; Whitt, M.A.; de la Torre, J.C.; Zinkernagel, R.M. Kinetics of protective antibodies are determined by the viral surface antigen. *J. Clin. Investig.* **2004**, *114*, 988–993. [CrossRef] [PubMed]
96. Wyatt, R.; Kwong, P.D.; Desjardins, E.; Sweet, R.W.; Robinson, J.; Hendrickson, W.A.; Sodroski, J.G. The antigenic structure of the hiv gp120 envelope glycoprotein. *Nature* **1998**, *393*, 705–711. [CrossRef] [PubMed]
97. Gristick, H.B.; von Boehmer, L.; West, A.P., Jr.; Schamber, M.; Gazumyan, A.; Golijanin, J.; Seaman, M.S.; Fatkenheuer, G.; Klein, F.; Nussenzweig, M.C.; et al. Natively glycosylated hiv-1 env structure reveals new mode for antibody recognition of the cd4-binding site. *Nat. Struct. Mol. Biol.* **2016**, *23*, 906–915. [CrossRef] [PubMed]
98. Burnett, D.L.; Langley, D.B.; Schofield, P.; Hermes, J.R.; Chan, T.D.; Jackson, J.; Bourne, K.; Reed, J.H.; Patterson, K.; Porebski, B.T.; et al. Germinal center antibody mutation trajectories are determined by rapid self/foreign discrimination. *Science* **2018**, *360*, 223–226. [CrossRef] [PubMed]
99. Cooke, M.P.; Heath, A.W.; Shokat, K.M.; Zeng, Y.; Finkelman, F.D.; Linsley, P.S.; Howard, M.; Goodnow, C.C. Immunoglobulin signal transduction guides the specificity of b cell-t cell interactions and is blocked in tolerant self-reactive b cells. *J. Exp. Med.* **1994**, *179*, 425–438. [CrossRef] [PubMed]

100. Zhao, M.; Chen, J.; Tan, S.; Dong, T.; Jiang, H.; Zheng, J.; Quan, C.; Liao, Q.; Zhang, H.; Wang, X.; et al. Prolonged evolution of virus-specific memory t cell immunity post severe avian influenza a (h7n9) virus infection. *J. Virol.* **2018**. [CrossRef] [PubMed]
101. Ping, X.; Hu, W.; Xiong, R.; Zhang, X.; Teng, Z.; Ding, M.; Li, L.; Chang, C.; Xu, K. Generation of a broadly reactive influenza h1 antigen using a consensus ha sequence. *Vaccine* **2018**, *36*, 4837–4845. [CrossRef] [PubMed]
102. Bachmann, M.F.; Rohrer, U.H.; Kundig, T.M.; Burki, K.; Hengartner, H.; Zinkernagel, R.M. The influence of antigen organization on b cell responsiveness. *Science* **1993**, *262*, 1448–1451. [CrossRef] [PubMed]
103. Ilyinskii, P.O.; Thoidis, G.; Sherman, M.Y.; Shneider, A. Adjuvant potential of aggregate-forming polyglutamine domains. *Vaccine* **2008**, *26*, 3223–3226. [CrossRef] [PubMed]
104. Van Braeckel-Budimir, N.; Haijema, B.J.; Leenhouts, K. Bacterium-like particles for efficient immune stimulation of existing vaccines and new subunit vaccines in mucosal applications. *Front. Immunol.* **2013**, *4*, 282. [CrossRef] [PubMed]
105. Snapper, C.M. Distinct immunologic properties of soluble versus particulate antigens. *Front. Immunol.* **2018**, *9*, 598. [CrossRef] [PubMed]
106. Strand, M.; August, J.T. Structural proteins of mammalian oncogenic rna viruses: Multiple antigenic determinants of the major internal protein and envelope glycoprotein. *J. Virol.* **1974**, *13*, 171–180. [PubMed]
107. Shubin, Z.; Li, W.; Poonia, B.; Ferrari, G.; LaBranche, C.; Montefiori, D.; Zhu, X.; Pauza, C.D. An hiv envelope gp120-fc fusion protein elicits effector antibody responses in rhesus macaques. *Clin. Vaccine Immunol.* **2017**, *24*, 00028-17. [CrossRef] [PubMed]
108. Robinson, J.E.; Hastie, K.M.; Cross, R.W.; Yenni, R.E.; Elliott, D.H.; Rouelle, J.A.; Kannadka, C.B.; Smira, A.A.; Garry, C.E.; Bradley, B.T.; et al. Most neutralizing human monoclonal antibodies target novel epitopes requiring both lassa virus glycoprotein subunits. *Nat. Commun.* **2016**, *7*, 11544. [CrossRef] [PubMed]
109. Provine, N.M.; Cortez, V.; Chohan, V.; Overbaugh, J. The neutralization sensitivity of viruses representing human immunodeficiency virus type 1 variants of diverse subtypes from early in infection is dependent on producer cell, as well as characteristics of the specific antibody and envelope variant. *Virology* **2012**, *427*, 25–33. [CrossRef] [PubMed]
110. Cohen, Y.Z.; Lorenzi, J.C.C.; Seaman, M.S.; Nogueira, L.; Schoofs, T.; Krassnig, L.; Butler, A.; Millard, K.; Fitzsimons, T.; Daniell, X.; et al. Neutralizing activity of broadly neutralizing anti-hiv-1 antibodies against clade b clinical isolates produced in peripheral blood mononuclear cells. *J. Virol.* **2018**, *92*, e01883-17. [PubMed]
111. Huang, J.; Kang, B.H.; Pancera, M.; Lee, J.H.; Tong, T.; Feng, Y.; Imamichi, H.; Georgiev, I.S.; Chuang, G.Y.; Druz, A.; et al. Broad and potent hiv-1 neutralization by a human antibody that binds the gp41-gp120 interface. *Nature* **2014**, *515*, 138–142. [CrossRef] [PubMed]
112. Leon, P.E.; He, W.; Mullarkey, C.E.; Bailey, M.J.; Miller, M.S.; Krammer, F.; Palese, P.; Tan, G.S. Optimal activation of fc-mediated effector functions by influenza virus hemagglutinin antibodies requires two points of contact. *Proc. Natl. Acad. Sci. USA* **2016**, *113*, E5944–E5951. [CrossRef] [PubMed]
113. Abreu-Mota, T.; Hagen, K.R.; Cooper, K.; Jahrling, P.B.; Tan, G.; Wirblich, C.; Johnson, R.F.; Schnell, M.J. Non-neutralizing antibodies elicited by recombinant lassa-rabies vaccine are critical for protection against lassa fever. *Nat. Commun.* **2018**, *9*, 4223. [CrossRef] [PubMed]
114. An, L.L.; Whitton, J.L. A multivalent minigene vaccine, containing b-cell, cytotoxic t-lymphocyte, and th epitopes from several microbes, induces appropriate responses in vivo and confers protection against more than one pathogen. *J. Virol.* **1997**, *71*, 2292–2302. [PubMed]
115. Holst, P.J.; Jensen, B.A.; Ragonnaud, E.; Thomsen, A.R.; Christensen, J.P. Targeting of non-dominant antigens as a vaccine strategy to broaden t-cell responses during chronic viral infection. *PLoS ONE* **2015**, *10*, e0117242. [CrossRef] [PubMed]
116. Rammensee, H.G.; Friede, T.; Stevanoviic, S. Mhc ligands and peptide motifs: First listing. *Immunogenetics* **1995**, *41*, 178–228. [CrossRef] [PubMed]
117. Patarroyo, M.E.; Bermudez, A.; Alba, M.P.; Vanegas, M.; Moreno-Vranich, A.; Poloche, L.A.; Patarroyo, M.A. Impips: The immune protection-inducing protein structure concept in the search for steric-electron and topochemical principles for complete fully-protective chemically synthesised vaccine development. *PLoS ONE* **2015**, *10*, e0123249. [CrossRef] [PubMed]

118. Lozano, J.M.; Varela, Y.; Silva, Y.; Ardila, K.; Forero, M.; Guasca, L.; Guerrero, Y.; Bermudez, A.; Alba, P.; Vanegas, M.; et al. A large size chimeric highly immunogenic peptide presents multistage plasmodium antigens as a vaccine candidate system against malaria. *Molecules* **2017**, *22*, 1837. [CrossRef] [PubMed]
119. Mukhopadhyay, M.; Galperin, M.; Patgaonkar, M.; Vasan, S.; Ho, D.D.; Nouel, A.; Claireaux, M.; Benati, D.; Lambotte, O.; Huang, Y.; et al. DNA vaccination by electroporation amplifies broadly cross-restricted public tcr clonotypes shared with hiv controllers. *J. Immunol.* **2017**, *199*, 3437–3452. [CrossRef] [PubMed]
120. Liu, F.; Feuer, R.; Hassett, D.E.; Whitton, J.L. Peptide vaccination of mice immune to lcmv or vaccinia virus causes serious cd8 t cell-mediated, tnf-dependent immunopathology. *J. C. Investig.* **2006**, *116*, 465–475. [CrossRef] [PubMed]
121. Sissoko, D.; Laouenan, C.; Folkesson, E.; M'Lebing, A.B.; Beavogui, A.H.; Baize, S.; Camara, A.M.; Maes, P.; Shepherd, S.; Danel, C.; et al. Experimental treatment with favipiravir for ebola virus disease (the jiki trial): A historically controlled, single-arm proof-of-concept trial in guinea. *PLoS Med.* **2016**, *13*, e1001967.
122. Kentsis, A.; Volpon, L.; Topisirovic, I.; Soll, C.E.; Culjkovic, B.; Shao, L.; Borden, K.L. Further evidence that ribavirin interacts with eif4e. *RNA* **2005**, *11*, 1762–1766. [CrossRef] [PubMed]
123. Volpon, L.; Culjkovic-Kraljacic, B.; Sohn, H.S.; Blanchet-Cohen, A.; Osborne, M.J.; Borden, K.L.B. A biochemical framework for eif4e-dependent mrna export and nuclear recycling of the export machinery. *RNA* **2017**, *23*, 927–937. [CrossRef] [PubMed]
124. Iwasaki, M.; de la Torre, J.C. A highly conserved leucine in mammarenavirus matrix z protein is required for z interaction with the virus l polymerase and z stability in cells harboring an active viral ribonucleoprotein. *J. Virol.* **2018**, *92*, 02256-17. [CrossRef] [PubMed]
125. Hickerson, B.T.; Westover, J.B.; Jung, K.H.; Komeno, T.; Furuta, Y.; Gowen, B.B. Effective treatment of experimental lymphocytic choriomeningitis virus infection: Consideration of favipiravir for use with infected organ transplant recipients. *J. Infect. Dis.* **2018**, *218*, 522–527. [CrossRef] [PubMed]

pathogens

MDPI

Article

Attenuated Replication of Lassa Virus Vaccine Candidate ML29 in STAT-1$^{-/-}$ Mice

Dylan M. Johnson [1,3,*], Jenny D. Jokinen [2,3] and Igor S. Lukashevich [2,3,*]

1 Department of Microbiology and Immunology, University of Louisville Health Sciences Center, Louisville, KY 40292, USA
2 Department of Pharmacology and Toxicology, University of Louisville Health Sciences Center, Louisville, KY 40292, USA; jenny.jokinen@louisville.edu
3 Center for Predictive Medicine for Biodefense and Emerging Infectious Diseases, NIH Regional Biocontainment Laboratory, Louisville, KY 40222, USA
* Correspondence: dylan.johnson@louisville.edu (D.M.J.); igor.lukashevich@louisville.edu (I.S.L.)

Received: 6 December 2018; Accepted: 11 January 2019; Published: 15 January 2019

Abstract: Lassa virus (LASV), a highly prevalent mammalian arenavirus endemic in West Africa, can cause Lassa fever (LF), which is responsible for thousands of deaths annually. LASV is transmitted to humans from naturally infected rodents. At present, there is not an effective vaccine nor treatment. The genetic diversity of LASV is the greatest challenge for vaccine development. The reassortant ML29 carrying the L segment from the nonpathogenic Mopeia virus (MOPV) and the S segment from LASV is a vaccine candidate under current development. ML29 demonstrated complete protection in validated animal models against a Nigerian strain from clade II, which was responsible for the worst outbreak on record in 2018. This study demonstrated that ML29 was more attenuated than MOPV in STAT1$^{-/-}$ mice, a small animal model of human LF and its sequelae. ML29 infection of these mice resulted in more than a thousand-fold reduction in viremia and viral load in tissues and strong LASV-specific adaptive T cell responses compared to MOPV-infected mice. Persistent infection of Vero cells with ML29 resulted in generation of interfering particles (IPs), which strongly interfered with the replication of LASV, MOPV and LCMV, the prototype of the Arenaviridae. ML29 IPs induced potent cell-mediated immunity and were fully attenuated in STAT1$^{-/-}$ mice. Formulation of ML29 with IPs will improve the breadth of the host's immune responses and further contribute to development of a pan-LASV vaccine with full coverage meeting the WHO requirements.

Keywords: Lassa virus vaccine; ML29 vaccine; STAT-1$^{-/-}$ mice; Lassa virus; Mopeia virus; interfering particles

1. Introduction

Lassa virus (LASV) is a highly prevalent arenavirus in West Africa, where it infects several hundred thousand individuals annually. This results in a large number of Lassa fever (LF) cases associated with high morbidity and mortality rates [1,2]. The natural LASV reservoir is the rodent *Mastomys natalensis*, which is widely distributed throughout sub-Saharan Africa. The area where LASV is endemic covers large regions of West Africa [3], putting a population of up to 200 million people at risk for infection [4]. Furthermore, there is evidence that LASV-endemic regions are expanding [5]. The high degree of LASV genetic diversity [6,7] likely contributes to underestimates of its prevalence [8]. With the exception of dengue fever, LF has the greatest estimated global burden among all viral hemorrhagic fevers (HFs) [9]. LF outbreaks are associated with mortality rates as high as 60%, as documented during the 2015–2016 outbreak in Nigeria [10]. The currently ongoing 2018 outbreak is the worst on record [11]. There is no FDA-approved LASV vaccine or therapeutic. Treatment options are limited to off-label ribavirin with varying degrees of success. In 2017–2018, the WHO included LASV on the top priority pathogens list and issued a Target Product Profile (TPP) for LASV vaccine development [12–14].

LASV belongs to the Old World (OW) group (former lymphocytic choriomeningitis virus, LCMV-LASV sero-complex) of the genus *Mammarenavirus* of the *Arenaviridae* family [15]. The LASV genome has two RNA segments that each encode two open reading frames in opposite polarities, separated by a structured intergenic region. The L-RNA encodes for a large L protein, which functions as a RNA-dependent RNA polymerase (RdRp), and a RING finger protein Z, which comprises the matrix of virions. The S-RNA encodes for a nucleoprotein (NP) which tightly associates with viral RNA and a glycoprotein precursor (GPC) that is processed into three subunits: a stable signal peptide, SSP; a receptor-binding GP1; and a transmembrane GP2, which mediates fusion with cell membranes. All three glycoprotein subunits associate to form club-shaped features on the surface of pleomorphic viral particles, which vary in the diameter from 50 to 300 nm. In addition to LASV, the OW group includes genetically related nonpathogenic viruses: Mopeia (MOPV), Morogoro (MORV), Gairo (GAIV) and Luna (LUNV) hosted by the same rodents [16–19]. The New World (NW) mammalian arenaviruses (former Tacaribe virus, TCRV, sero-complex) comprise viruses that circulate in the Americas, and include the causative agents of South American HFs [20].

Reassortant studies using genetically related mammalian arenaviruses with different pathogenic potential demonstrated that the L gene is responsible for high levels of virus replication in vivo, and is associated with acute disease in experimental animals [21,22]. Coinfection of cells with LASV and MOPV resulted in generation of MOPV/LASV reassortants [23,24]. One of the rationally selected clones, ML29, carrying the L-RNA from MOPV and the S-RNA from the Josiah strain of LASV (LASV/JOS), is a promising LASV vaccine candidate [24–26].

While MOPV L-RNA is the major driving force of ML29 attenuation, 18 mutations incorporated in the ML29 genome during in vitro selection additionally seem to contribute to the attenuation of ML29 [25,27]. Indeed, transcriptome profiling of human peripheral blood mononuclear cells (hPBMC) exposed to LASV or ML29 exhibited distinct molecular signatures that can be useful biomarkers of pathogenicity and protection [28,29]. Similar studies comparing MOPV and ML29 infected hPBMC revealed that gene expression patterns in mock and ML29 infected hPBMC clustered together and differed from the expression pattern observed in MOPV infected hPBMC [28].

Recently, recombinant ML29 (rML29) was rescued from cDNA clones and demonstrated the same features as a biological ML29 (bML29) [30]. Reverse genetics provides a powerful tool for elucidation of the individual contributions of ML29-specific mutations to attenuation. However, the absence of a reliable small animal model for LASV pathogenicity is a major obstacle for the field. LASV, as well as other mammalian arenaviruses, stimulate antiviral immunity differently in natural rodent hosts and in humans and non-human primates, NHPs [31–33]. While some pathogenic features of human LF can be observed in strain 13 guinea pigs [34–36], there is a poor correlation between clinical outcome of LF in humans and virulence of LASV in guinea pigs [37]. Results of LASV vaccination/challenge studies in strain 13 guinea pigs are not reproducible in NHPs [32,38,39]. In addition, strain 13 guinea pigs are no longer commercially available and difficult to breed.

Rodent models remain useful to study some mechanisms of LF pathogenesis and protective immune responses, and to provide valuable information during preclinical development of vaccine candidates [31,40]. Previous research has documented that mice lacking a functional STAT1 pathway are highly susceptible to LASV infection, and develop fatal disease with some pathological features that mimic human LF [41]. Notably, human LASV isolates from fatal LF cases in Sierra Leone induced clinically similar fatal disease including high viral load in blood and visceral organs of STAT-1$^{-/-}$ mice after intraperitoneal inoculation (i.p.). In contrast, LASV isolated from a non-lethal human case induced disease with moderate mortality. Surviving mice developed hearing loss that mimicked the sensorineural hearing loss (SNHL) commonly observed in LF patients during convalescence [42].

In this study, we provided additional evidence of deep ML29 attenuation by modeling the LASV infection protocol for STAT$^{-/-}$ mice as a means to assess the safety profile of ML29 (bML29 or rML29) in comparison with MOPV. We also generated ML29 stocks enriched with interfering particles (IPs) produced by ML29-persisitently infected cells. The growing body of evidence indicates that, during natural infection, IPs are critically involved in the modulation of viral load, innate immune responses, disease outcome, and contribute to the evolutionary persistence of viruses [43–45]. An accumulation of IPs with genome deletions has been documented during the production of live-attenuated polio [46], influenza [47,48] and measles [49–51] vaccines, and was associated with modulating vaccine potency and immunostimulatory properties. Here, we demonstrated that STAT$^{-/-}$ mice are a susceptible model capable of discriminating between viruses with different levels of attenuation, MOPV and ML29. ML29 IPs were completely attenuated in these mice, enhancing immunogenic features of ML29. The broad cross-protection activity of ML29 IPs and their intrinsic adjuvant features can be potentially used for rational formulation of a pan-LASV ML29-based vaccine by developing vaccine-manufacturing protocols to optimize the ratio between infectious ML29 and IPs.

2. Results

2.1. Generation of Interfering Particles (IPs) by ML29-Persisitently Infected Cells

Arenavirus IPs can be generated at high multiplicity of infection (MOI) by serial infection of fresh tissue cultures with undiluted culture medium harvested from previous passages. Alternatively, initially infected cells can be subjected to serial passages. Both methods resulted in the accumulation of IPs. Earlier studies suggested a contribution of IPs in the establishment and/or maintenance of LCMV persistent infection in vitro and in vivo, and in the inhibition of virus-induced immunopathology in mice [52–58]. The protocol previously applied for the generation of LASV IPs in cell cultures was used to establish ML29 persistent infection of Vero cells. In line with previous observations [59–61], passages of ML29-infected cells, either infected with bML29 or with rML29, resulted in the gradual decline of infectious particles released in culture medium. As seen in Figure 1, the infectious titers of ML29 released into the medium of persistently infected Vero cells (Vero/ML29) were reduced almost 100-fold after 10 passages, and was under detectable levels after 15 passages. Vero/ML29 cells strongly interfered with replication of homologous (ML29) or genetically related LASV/JOS, LCMV, and MOPV and did not generate infectious plaques after super infection of Vero/ML29 with these viruses. Meanwhile, neither the replication of TCRV, a NW arenavirus, nor the nonrelated Ebola virus, was affected in these cells. ML29 IPs released from persistently infected Vero/ML29 cells were able to suppress replication of homologous virus in a dose-dependent manner (Figure 1f).

While the replication of ML29 or LASV was not detectable in ML29/Vero cells after passage 10, viral proteins were detected in these cells by immunofocus (IF) assay (Figure 1c). In contrast to infectious "plaques", this assay detects cells expressing virus antigens stained by specific antibodies. With an increasing number of passages, ML29-infected cells lost their ability to produce plaques after homologous superinfection, but were strongly positive for ML29-specific antigens as demonstrated by quantitated analyses (Figure 1c; Appendix A, Figure A1). Differences in the morphology of IF foci between naïve and Vero/ML29 cells after infection and superinfection with ML29, respectively, seems to be related to differences in the expression of NP and GP proteins in different passages of Vero/ML29 (Appendix A, Figure A1F).

The viral RNA load in Vero/ML29 cells, as assessed by quantitative qRT-PCR targeting the NP gene, declined about tenfold during the first five passages and persisted approximately at the same levels during subsequent passages of Vero/ML29 (Figure 1b). The viral RNA load remained at a similar level through 50 passages (data not shown). Our attempts failed to detect genomic RNA deletions using RT-PCR, either in infected cells or in virions released from infected cells (not shown, see Discussion).

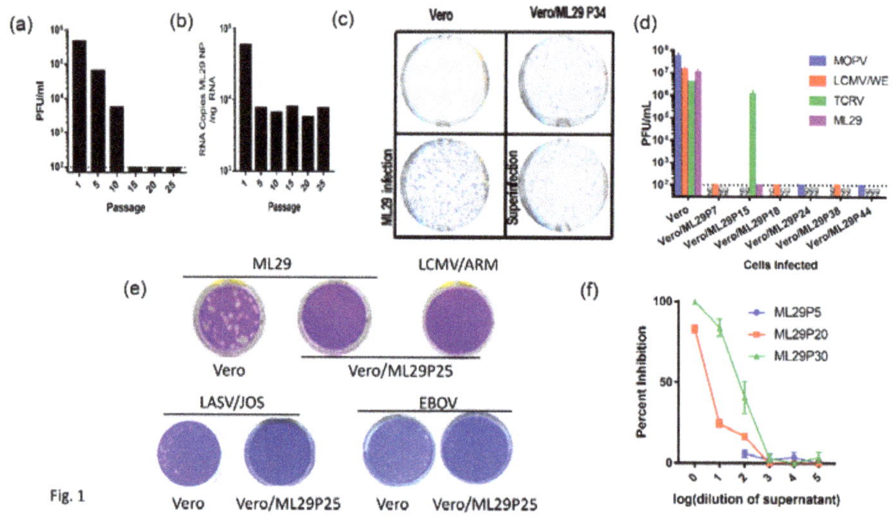

Figure 1. Vero cells persistently infected with ML29 interfere with replication of homologous and genetically related arenaviruses. (**a**) Supernatants from a Vero cell line persistently infected with ML29 (Vero/ML29) were titrated for infectious virus by plaque assay at the indicated passages. (**b**) Total RNA was isolated from a Vero/ML29 cells at the indicated passages and was assayed using qRT-PCR with a LASV/JOS nucleoprotein (NP) TaqMan probe. Copy number was determined by regression against a standard curve. (**c**) Immunofocus assay using polyclonal moneky-anti-ML29 on uninfected Vero E6 cells (top left), Vero/ML29 passage 34 cells (top right), Vero E6 cells infected with a 0.1 MOI of ML29 for 3 days (bottom left), and Vero/ML29 passage 34 cells superinfected with a 0.1 MOI of ML29 for 3 days (bottom right). (**d**) Naïve or persistently infected Vero/ML29 cells at different passages were used to titer MOPV, LCMV/WE, TCRV, ML29 by plaque assay. (**e**) Plaque-forming activity of Vero/ML29 cells. ML29 (top left and top center), LCMV/ARM (top right), LASV/JOS (bottom left and bottom left center), and EBOV (bottom right center and bottom right) were used in a plaque assay on Vero E6 cell (top left, bottom left, and bottom right center) or the 25th passage of a Vero cell line persistently infected with ML29, Vero/ML29P25 (top center, top right, bottom center left, bottom right.) (**f**) Dose-dependent effects of IPs on replication of ML29. Vero E6 cells were pre-incubated for 1 h with the indicated dilution of ML29 IPs produced by Vero/ML29 cells at passage 5, 20 or 30. The pretreated cells were then infected with standard ML29 and viral titer was determined by plaque assay. Percent inhibition is normalized to infectious titer determined on Vero E6 cells that were not pretreated.

2.2. MOPV and Attenuated Reassortant ML29 Induce Experimental Disease with Different Clinical Manifestations and Outcome in STAT-1$^{-/-}$ Mice

In STAT1$^{-/-}$ mice, LASV infection resulted in experimental disease with the outcome depending on the pathogenic potential of the LASV isolate [42]. Based on these observations, we tested the attenuation of MOPV and ML29 in these mice. Using the LASV infection protocol, three groups of mice (n = 9) were IP inoculated with MOPV, ML29 and ML29P50 (IPs produced by Vero/ML29, passage 50). MOPV infection resulted in poor grooming, lethargy and signs of dehydration starting around day 8-post-infection. These symptoms aggravated, and the mice gradually lost weight, and experienced a drop in body temperature. All animals in this group met euthanasia criteria within 11–17 days following infection (Figure 2). In ML29 infected STAT1$^{-/-}$ mice, the symptoms started to improve at the late stage of the infection. Body temperature quickly recovered after day 10 and 33% of mice survived at day 21. No clinical signs were observed in the ML29P50 group. These mice gained weight at the end of the observation period and their temperature fluctuated within a normal range.

As a control, wild-type mice with an identical genetic background were i.p. inoculated with MOPV, ML29 and ML29P50. The mice were successfully infected with these viruses as was documented by detection of viral RNA in tested tissues (Appendix A, Figure A2). However, in the wild-type mice, the replication of the viruses was well-controlled and viral RNA was barely detectable at day 21. As expected, infection did not induce clinical manifestations in any of the wild-type study groups, and these mice gained weight at the end of the 21-day observation period.

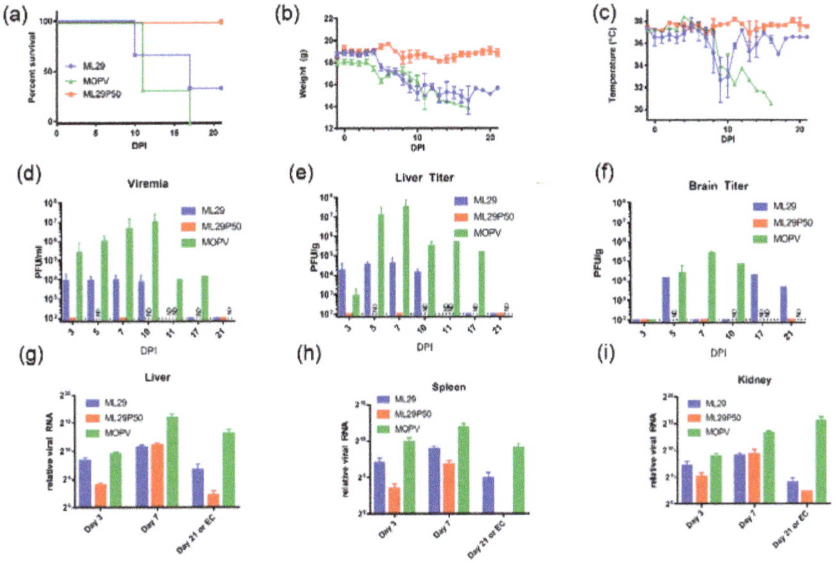

Figure 2. Clinical manifestation and outcome of MOPV and ML29 infections in STAT-1$^{-/-}$ mice. (**a**) Mice were infected (i.p.) with 1×10^3 PFU of MOPV An20410, ML29 (standard infectious virus) or with ML29P50 (IPs collected from culture medium of Vero/ML29P50 cells). ML29P50 IPs were quantified by MOPV L gene qRT-PCR and used in genome-equivalent dose, 1×10^3 PFU. (**b**) Weight and (**c**) Temperature of infected mice. (**d**) Viremia, (**e**) Infectious viral load in liver, and (**f**) brain of STAT-1$^{-/-}$ mice. (**g–i**) Viral RNA load assessed as relative expression of MOPV-L gene by qRT-PCR in the indicated tissues at the time point indicated. DPI, days post-infection. EC, endpoint criteria.

2.3. Replication of MOPV and ML29 in Tissues of STAT-$^{-/-}$ Mice: No Viremia and Infectious Virus in Tissues of ML29P50-Infected Mice

High viremia, infectious titers, and viral RNA loads were associated with replication of MOPV in tissues of STAT-1$^{-/-}$ mice as assessed by infectious plaque assay and qRT-PCR (Figure 2). At the peak of clinical manifestation, days 7–10, viremia and viral load in the liver reached more than 1×10^7 PFU/mL or PFU/g, respectively. RNAscope in situ hybridization confirmed extensive liver infection with strong signals associated with hepatocytes and endothelial cells (Figure 3, arrowed). In contrast, replication of ML29 was more attenuated in STAT-1$^{-/-}$ mice. Viremia and viral load in the liver was 3-logs lower in these mice compared with MOPV infection, and only a few weakly positive hepatocytes were seen in ML29-infected liver samples. In brain tissue, replication of infectious ML29 was transiently detected at early and late stages of infection. Replication of infectious ML29P50 in STAT-1$^{-/-}$ mice was below detectable levels in blood, liver and brain. However, replication of ML29P50 was detected in tissues by viral RNA-based assays, qRT-PCR, and RNAscope in situ hybridization. As seen in Figure 2g–i, at early stage of the infection, relative levels of ML29P50 viral RNA in tissues were lower than MOPV and ML29 viral RNAs. ML29P50 was barely detectable in the tissues at late stage of the infection.

This indicates that ML29P50 was well-controlled, an observation that is in line with the absence of clinical manifestations.

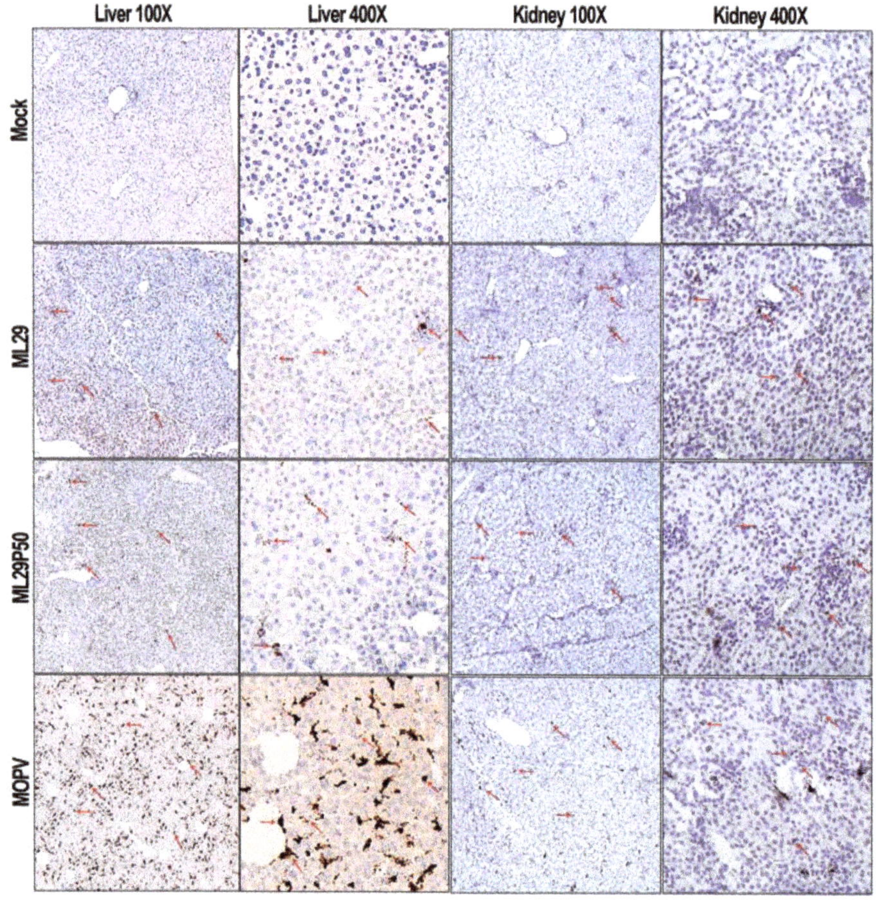

Figure 3. RNAscope in situ hybridization. Representative images at two different magnifications (100× and 400×) of RNAscope in situ hybridization (brown spots, arrowed) targeting the MOPV-L gene in the liver and kidney of STAT1$^{-/-}$ mice.

2.4. Host Responses in Mice Infected with MOPV and ML29

Cell-mediated immune responses in infected mice were assessed by ELISPOT using stimulation of spleen cells isolated on day 3, 7, and 21 after infection with peptide cocktails derived from LASV/JOS GPC and MOPV GPC as previously described [62,63]. At day 3, virus-specific T cells secreting IFN-γ, IL-2 or both were barely detectable in all groups of mice (not shown). By day 7, in STAT-1$^{-/-}$ mice, comparable levels of IFN-γ-secreting cells (~0.4% of total spleen cells) were observed in spleens from ML29- and ML29P50-infected mice (Figure 4a). In wild-type mice, ML29 and ML29P50 infection induced slightly lower T-cell responses Notably, in wild-type and STAT-1$^{-/-}$ mice infected either with ML29 or with ML29P50, similar levels of IFN-γ-secreting cells were induced after stimulation with GPC cocktails derived from LASV or MOPV. Infection with MOPV induced comparatively diminished T cell responses in wild-type and in STAT-1$^{-/-}$ mice, predominantly after stimulation with homologous MOPV GPC-derived peptides. After stimulation with GPC cocktails, spleen cells isolated from mice infected with ML29 and ML29P50, but not with MOPV, also secreted IL-2 cytokine, ~0.1% of total spleen cells. Cells secreting both cytokines were easily detectable at day 7 in ML29 and ML29P50 mice after stimulation with homologous antigens. In MOPV infected STAT-1$^{-/-}$ mice, this cells population was barely detectable.

Survival of ML29P50-infected mice was clearly associated with strong cell-mediated responses. As seen in Figure 4, in spleens isolated from STAT-1$^{-/-}$ mice on day 21, cells secreting IFN-γ, IL2, or both were strongly upregulated after stimulation with GPC cocktails, >0.3–0.6%. In wild-type mice inoculated with ML29P50, these responses had declined by this time point. Interestingly enough, in both groups of mice infected with ML29P50 humoral responses were similar (Figure 4g).

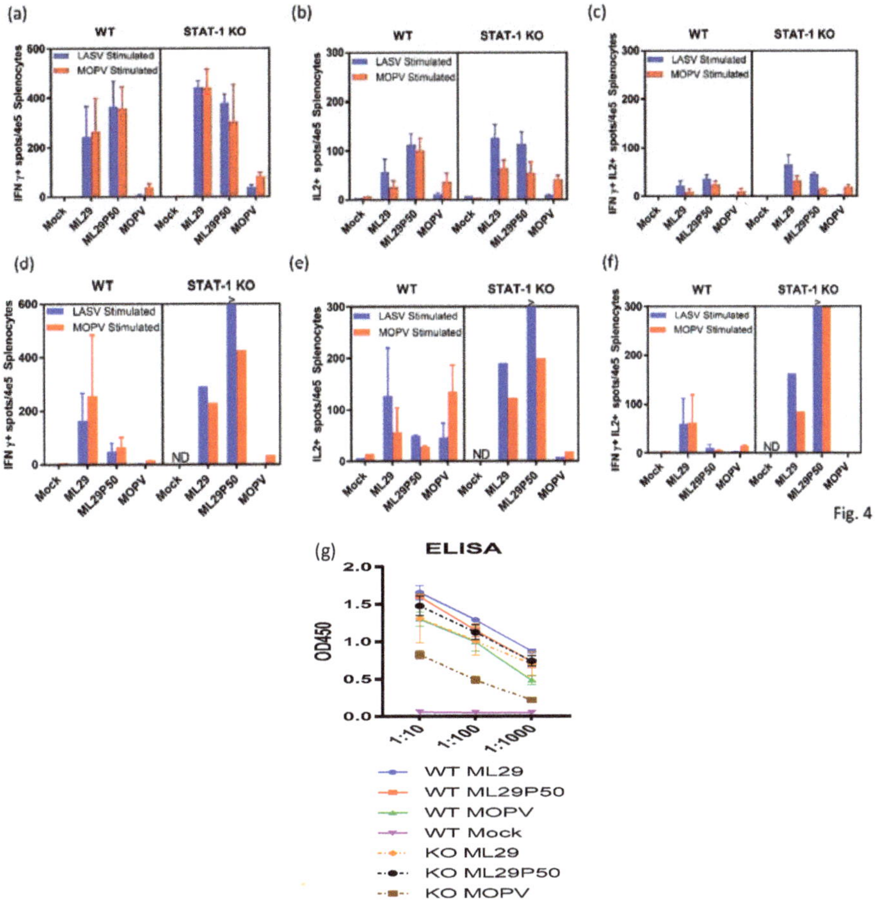

Figure 4. Adaptive immune responses of STAT-1$^{-/-}$ mice. ELISPOT counts per 4×10^5 splenocytes from STAT-1$^{-/-}$ mice or wild-type (WT) controls collected (**a–c**) 7 days post-infection or (**d–f**) at endpoint criteria or 21 days post-infection. Splenocytes were stimulated with LASV GPC or MOPV GPC-derived peptide cocktails for 24 h. (**a**,**d**) IFN-γ-secreted cells, (**b**,**e**) IL-2-secreted cells, or (**c**,**d**) poly-functional IFN-γ/IL-2-secreting cells. (**g**) Antibody responses measured by IgG ELISA in the serum of STAT-1$^{-/-}$ mice or wild-type controls collected at 21 days post-infection or endpoint criteria. >, Too numerous to count.

Measurement of pro-inflammatory cytokine expression in spleen of STAT-1$^{-/-}$ mice infected with MOPV revealed upregulation of IL-6 and IL-1β at early stages of the infection and rapidly declined at later time points while TNF-α was downregulated for all viruses except the early stages of MOPV and the late stage of ML29P50 (Figure 5, Appendix A, Figure A3). Levels of IL-1β and IL-6 mRNA in spleens of the mice infected with ML29 and ML25P50 were upregulated at day 3 and day 7, respectively. At the later time point, the infection had minimal if any effect on TNF-α and IL-1β expression in STAT-1$^{-/-}$ and control mice. In MOPV-infected wild-type mice, IL-6 mRNA levels had similar kinetics with those in STAT-1$^{-/-}$ mice, with downregulation in the liver and spleen tissues during the infection.

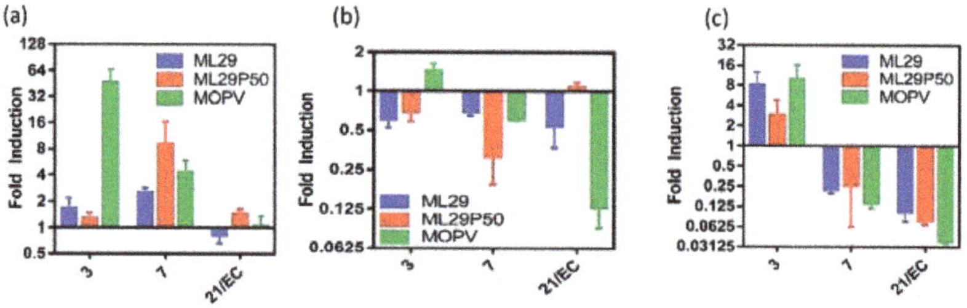

Figure 5. Cytokine responses of STAT-1$^{-/-}$ mice. (**a**) IL-6, (**b**) TNF-α, or (**c**) IL-1β expression in splenocytes of STAT-1$^{-/-}$ mice relative to mock infected by qRT-PCR.

3. Discussion

The first aim of this study was to determine if STAT-1$^{-/-}$ mice provide a reliable small animal model to assess level of attenuation of LASV-related arenaviruses. LASV and MOPV share a common reservoir, *M. natalensis*, found in the western and southeastern regions of Africa [16,17,64]. In Mozambique and Tanzania, areas where MOPV and MORV are prevalent, there is a marked absence of clinical cases of LF. Additionally, MOPV does not cause clinical signs in guinea pigs and NHPs [35]. These observations, combined with ability of MOPV to generate in vitro replication-competent reassortants with LASV [24], and to protect experimentally infected NHPs against fatal LF [65], suggests that MOPV is a "naturally attenuated" genetic relative of LASV.

Studies to assess virulence of human LASV isolates in NHPs are very limited [66]. LASV isolates from LF patients with different clinical outcome showed a weak correlation between severity of human disease and virulence in guinea pigs [35,37]. Meanwhile, in STAT-1$^{-/-}$ mice, outcome of the disease correlated with virulence of human LASV isolates. Four out of 5 mice infected with a lethal isolate met euthanasia criteria between days 7 and 8, while mice infected with nonlethal LASV isolates developed chronic disease [41,42]. In our experiments, MOPV infection of STAT-1$^{-/-}$ mice induced manifested disease that met euthanasia criteria 11–17 days post-infection (Figure 2a). The delayed euthanasia time-point of 11–17 days versus 7–8 days indicates some level of attenuation of MOPV infection in STAT-1$^{-/-}$ mice. However, high levels of viremia and viral load in target tissues, comparable with those in animals infected with virulent LASV isolates [41,42], and poor adaptive immune responses (Figure 4) resulted in aggravated disease. In contrast to MOPV, ML29 infection in STAT-1$^{-/-}$ mice was more attenuated, and 33% of animals survived in this group (Figure 2a). Compared to MOPV-infected mice, ML29 infection notably resulted in more than a thousand-fold reduction in viremia and viral load in tissues by plaque assay (Figure 2d–f). Strong T cell responses contributed to viral control in this experimental group (Figure 4). It is well documented that strong T cell-mediated immunity correlates with protection and positive clinical outcomes in experimentally infected NHPs and LF patients [33,67–69].

The second aim of this study was to assess the contribution of IPs generated by ML29-persistently infected cells to the attenuation and modulation of immune responses. Similar to many other RNA viruses, mammalian arenaviruses can generate IPs during acute infection of cells at high MOI, or during persistent infection. The defective IPs: (i) are antigenically identical to parental viruses and contain the same structural proteins; (ii) preserve 5′ and 3′ terminal sequences of parental genome but have extensive internal deletions; (iii) can only replicate with help of standard virus; and (iv) strongly compete for replication machinery with the parental virus [70–74]. Historically, arenavirus IPs were observed following in vitro infection at high MOI, and masked the cell-killing potential of standard viruses. Earlier studies suggested the contribution of IPs in the establishment and/or maintenance of LCMV persistent infection in vitro, and in inhibition of virus-induced immunopathology in mice [52–58]. Similarly, LASV IPs generated by persistently infected cells strongly interfered with replication of standard LASV in vitro, were attenuated in C3H mice, and partially protected mice against wild-type LASV challenge [59,60,75,76]. In contrast to IPs generated from VSV, Sendai, Sindbis, and other RNA viruses, arenavirus IPs are difficult to separate from standard virions [55]. The unique ability of mammalian arenaviruses to incorporate host ribosomes and RNAs during the late stage of virus maturation [15] seems to be responsible for failure of density-based methods to purify arenavirus IPs. Nevertheless, LCMV defective IPs partially purified from culture medium of persistently infected cells lacked the S-RNA segment [77], compared to LASV defective IPs where the L RNA segment was not detectable [61]. In line with these results, UV inactivation experiments confirmed "smaller" genomes for LCMV [54] and LASV defective IPs [61]. The LCMV L-RNA segment was much less abundant and not detectable during the early stage of persistent infection. However, RNA deletions were not found among virus-specific RNA species in brain tissue of LCMV persistently infected mice. During the progression of persistence, an accumulation of terminally truncated RNA species was documented [78].

In our experiments, we were able to demonstrate the basic features of ML29 IPs generated by persistently infected cells (gradual infectivity loss during passages, antigenic identity and persistence, GP/NP ratio fluctuation, interference with homologous and closely related viruses) (Appendix A, Figure A1). However, we failed to detect genomic deletions among virus-specific RNA species extracted from persistently infected cells or among viral RNA extracted from concentrated supernatants by RT-PCR methods using different sets of primers to amplify the genomic L and S RNA segments. By using qRT-PCR quantification of the LASV(ML29) NP gene, we demonstrated that S-RNA copies rapidly declined during the first five cell culture passages of infected cells and the number of copies persisted at roughly same levels during passages 10–25 (Figure 1b). These levels remain relatively constant for all subsequent passages tested through passage 50 (not shown). In contrast to the permanent level of the S-RNA replication and protein expression detected by IF assay (Figure 1d), the infectivity of particles produced by persistently infected cells dropped dramatically during the first 10 passages, was below the threshold of detection by passage 15 (Figure 1a), and was not detectable at the final passage 50.

The inability of ML29-persistently infected cells to generate infectious plaques after homologous superinfection with ML29, or infection with LASV/JOS or MOPV, can be partially explained by arenavirus Z-mediated "superinfection exclusion" [79]. However, the replication of the NW mammalian arenavirus TCRV was not affected in ML29/Vero cells (Figure 1f). Recent study documented the capability of LCMV, LASV and MACV mammalian arenaviruses to replicate and disseminate without the Z protein providing evidence that NP can play role as potential surrogate of the Z protein [80]. We assume that ML29 IPs-induced interference was unlikely to be related to Z protein. Nevertheless, the contribution of the Z protein to innate immune responses cannot be fully excluded. ML29 has Z protein derived from MOPV. Interestingly enough, Z protein of pathogenic arenaviruses (including LASV,) but not that of nonpathogenic viruses, including the MOPV Z, inhibit RIG-I-like receptor-dependent IFN type I production [81].

In this study, we failed to provide evidence that ML29 IPs produced by ML29/Vero cells are "classical" defective IPs and the nature of ML29 IP-based interference has to be further elucidated. Nevertheless, ML29 IPs seem to be very attractive for vaccine formulation and development. First, as seen in Figure 2a, ML29P50 generated by ML29/Vero cells, passage 50, were completely attenuated in STAT-1$^{-/-}$ mice. These particles were not detectable by plaque assay (test on infectivity) in blood and tissues of mice. However, the level of ML29P50 RNA replication was similar or only slightly reduced in comparison with "wild-type" ML29 RNA replication (Figure 2g–i). Second, while ML29P50 and ML29 induced comparable T cell responses at day 7, at the late stage of the infection ML29P50 generated much stronger T cell immunity as assessed by IFN-γ/IL-2 ELISPOT in line with the strong immunomodulation potency of defective IPs [82]. While the mechanism of LASV protection can be dependent on the vaccine platform itself, as well as the animal challenge protocol—in the case of the ML29 vaccine, T cell immunity, but not antibody production—was associated with protection of NHPs [83]. Third, ML29 is the only vaccine with documented evidence of T-cell-mediated cross-protection against Nigerian LASV strains from clade II, among currently available LASV vaccine candidates [84]. This is critical considering the Nigerian LASV strains from clade II are responsible for causing the current unprecedented LF outbreak. LASV genetic diversity is the greatest challenge for vaccine development. The formulation of ML29 with IPs will improve the breadth of the host's immune responses [85] and further contribute to the development of a pan-LASV vaccine with full coverage meeting the WHO requirements [13].

4. Materials and Methods

4.1. *Viruses and Cells*

Generation of MOPV An20410, LASV/Josiah, and MOP/LAS reassortant (ML29) LCMV (WE and ARM) stocks in Vero cells and plaque titration technique was previously described [25]. Freeze-dried Tacaribe virus (TCRV-11573, ATCC® VR-1272CAF™) was purchased from ATCC and the virus stock was prepared by low MOI passage in Vero cells. Infectious plaques for all viruses, except MOPV, were counted at 5 days after infection by treatment of infected cell monolayers under agarose overlay with 4% paraformaldehyde and staining with 1% crystal violet. For MOPV, neutral red stain staining was used for plaque development. Vero C1008 cells (Vero 76, clone E6, ATCC® CRL1586) were maintained in DMEM/F-12 supplemented with 10% fetal calf serum, 1X antibiotic-antimycotic (ThermoFisher), and 1X Glutamax (ThermoFisher). ML29 persistent infection in Vero cells was established by using a previously described protocol [59,61]. In brief, after the initial infection of Vero cell monolayers with an MOI of 1.0, at weekly intervals, cells were detached from cell tissue flasks by treatment with 0.05% trypsin-EDTA (ThermoFisher) and subcultured at a 1:10 ratio. Culture medium was changed at 3–4-day intervals. Samples of cells and/or culture medium were used for plaque titration, antigen detection assays (IF, Western) and for RNA isolation. To titrate ML29 IPs produced by persistently infected Vero/ML29 cells, monolayers of naïve Vero cells were pretreated with dilutions of Vero/ML29 passage 5, 20 and 30 supernatants for 1 h followed by infection with ML29 and detection of plaques as described above. LASV/JOS or EBOV plaque titrations were performed in BSL-4 facilities using maximum containment practices at the University of Texas Medical Branch with the assistance of Dr. Slobodan Paessler's lab.

4.2. *Immunofocus Assay*

Vero E6 cells or ML29 persistently infected cells (Vero/ML29) were plated at a density of 2×10^4 cells/well in 96-well tissue culture plates. Twenty-four hours later, cells were overlaid with methylcellulose media. Naïve or Vero/ML29 cells were infected with 0.1 MOI of ML29 for 1 h prior to being overlaid with methylcellulose. After 3 days, the methylcellulose was removed and cells were then fixed with an acetone methanol mixture. Residual endogenous peroxidase was blocked by hydrogen peroxide and cells were incubated overnight in 10% FBS. After washing, cells were treated with either polyclonal monkey-anti-ML29 antibody (1:400), monoclonal mouse-anti-LASV/JOS-NP, 1:100 (GenScript, Piscataway, NJ, USA) or polyclonal rabbit-anti-LASV-GP 1:400 (IBT Bioservices, Rockville, MD, USA) followed by HRP linked appropriate secondary antibody. TrueBlue Peroxidase Substrate (SeraCare, Milford, MA, USA) was used for detection. Quantification of staining from high-quality images of scanned plates was performed using Adobe Photoshop to reduce background and threshold images followed by ImageJ counting of pixels.

4.3. Animal Protocols

Four-to-five week-old female STAT-1$^{-/-}$ mice (129S6/SvEv-Stat1tm1Rds) and wild-type controls (129SVE-F) were purchased from Taconic (Hudson, NY, USA). During a 1-week acclimation, a temperature and identification transponder was implanted subcutaneously and the mice were transferred to ABSL-3 housing at the NIH Regional Biocontainment Laboratory on the University of Louisville campus. For infection, 1×10^3 PFU of MOPV, ML29 or ML29P50 (quantitated as a qRT-PCR equivalent dose) was administered (i.p.) in 100 μL of PBS. Mice were monitored daily during 21 days and any animal with 25% weight loss was determined to have met the humane euthanasia criteria. Plasma samples from infected mice that had been euthanized were collected in EDTA tubes (BD). Tissue sample homogenates (10% *w*/*v*) were prepared with an Omni TH Tissue Homogenizer in DMEM/F12 followed with centrifugation at 4500× *g* for 20 min. Clarified tissue homogenates were tested in the plaque assay described above. All animal protocols were approved by the University of Louisville Institutional Animal Care and Use Committee.

4.4. qRT-PCR and RNAscope In Situ Hybridization

Tissue samples were placed into 2-mL screw-top tubes with 1 mL TRIzol Reagent (ThermoFisher) and glass beads, processed in a bead homogenizer, and tissue homogenates were stored at −80 °C until RNA isolation by phenol-chloroform extraction and ethanol precipitation. The qScript cDNA super mix (Quanta Biosciences) was used to make cDNA with an input of 1000 ng of RNA. qRT-PCR with TaqMan primers targeting the MOPV L gene, the LASV NP gene, IL-6, TNF-α, or IL-1β were used with a 18S housekeeping probe on a StepOnePlus qRT-PCR analyzer (Applied Biosystems). All IL-6, TNF-α, IL-1β and 18S primer/probe sets were commercially purchased through ThermoFisher Scientific through the Applied Biosystems division. Primer/probe set for MOPV amplified a region of the L segment (FWD 5′-TCCTCAATTAGG CGTGTGAA-3′; REV 5′-TACACATCCTTGGGTCCTGA-3′; probe 6FAM-CCCTGTTCCCTCCAACTTGTTCTT TG-TAMRA). Primer/probe set for LASV (ML29) amplified the NP gene segment (FWD 5′-TCC AACATATTGCCACCATC-3′; REV 5′- GCT GAC TCA AAG TCA TCC CA-3′; probe 6FAM TGCCTTCACAGCTGCACCCA-TAMRA). The qRT-PCR reaction contained 5 μM of each primer and 2 μM of probe for each primer/probe set, 5 μL of cDNA and TaqMan Fast Advanced Master Mix (ThermoFisher) in a final reaction volume of 20 μL. The reaction conditions were as follows: 50 °C for 2 min, 95 °C for 20 s then 40 cycles alternating between 95 °C for 3 s and 60 °C for 30 s. For RNAscope hybridization, fixed tissue sections were embedding in paraffin, cut on a Leica RM2125 RTS microtome, and mounted on glass slides. Custom designed target probes, preamplifier, amplifier, and label probe targeting MOPV L RNA were synthesized by Adanced Cell Diagnostics (Hayward, CA, USA) and RNAscope assay was performed according to the manufacturer's manual. Chromogenic detection was performed using DAB followed by counterstaining with hematoxylin.

4.5. EISPOT and IgG ELISA

Assessment of T cell responses in infected mice by the murine IFN-γ/IL-2 Double-Color Enzymatic ELISPOT (Cellular Technology Ltd., Cleveland, OH, USA) has been recently described [63]. In brief, erythrocyte-free splenocytes were added to 96-well filter plates (Millipore, MSIPS4510) pre-coated with anti-mouse cytokine antibody in triplicate at a density of 4×10^5 cells/well. Cells were stimulated overnight at 37 °C with cocktails of 10 μM LASV/JOS or MOPV GPC peptides (Mimotopes Ltd, Melbourne, Australia). Each cocktail contained 69 overlapping 20-mer peptides. As positive and negative controls, Conconavalin A (ThermoFisher) and CLT media alone was added to quality control wells. After stimulation, plates were developed according to the manufacturer's protocol and cells secreting individual cytokines IFN-γ or IL-2 or both were counted using C.T.L. Ltd. Immunospot® S5 Micro-analyzer and Immunospot® V 4.0 software. Quality control analysis was provided by C.T.L. Ltd.

IgG ELISA was performed as previously described [62]. In brief, microtiter plates were coated with 5 × 10^6 PFU/well of sonicated virus suspension in carbonate buffer (Sigma) overnight. Plates were washed, blocked with 10% milk for 2 h, washed again, and coated with dilutions of mouse serum for 1 h. Plates were washed and secondary HRP linked rabbit-anti-mouse IgG (Sigma) was added at a 1:2500 dilution for 1 h. Plates were washed and SureBlue TMB peroxidase substrate (SeraCare) was added for 15 min before the addition of TMB Stop Solution (SeraCare).

4.6. Statistics Analysis

Results are reported as means ± SEM (n = 4–5). ANOVA with Bonferroni's post-hoc test (for parametric data) or the Mann–Whitney rank-sum test (for nonparametric data) was used for the determination of statistical significance among treatment groups, as appropriate. Statistical analysis (mean, SD, T-test) and graphics were performed using the GraphPad Prism version 7 for Windows package (GraphPad Software, LaJolla, CA, USA).

Author Contributions: Conceptualization, I.S.L.; Methodology, I.S.L., D.M.J., J.D.J.; Animal Studies, D.M.J., J.D.J.; Data Analysis, I.S.L., D.M.J., J.D.J.; Visualization, D.M.J., J.D.J.; Writing, I.S.L., D.M.J.; Funding Acquisition, I.S.L.; Supervision, I.S.L.

Funding: This work was supported by grants R01AI093450 and R56AI135770 from the National Institute of Allergy and Infectious Diseases.

Acknowledgments: We thank the University of Louisville Center for Predictive Medicine for Biodefense and Emerging Infectious Diseases for the support of animal studies as well as Dr. Slobodan Paessler (The University of Texas Medical Branch at Galveston) for titration of Lassa and Ebola samples using Vero/ML29 cells.

Conflicts of Interest: The authors declare no conflicts of interest.

Appendix A

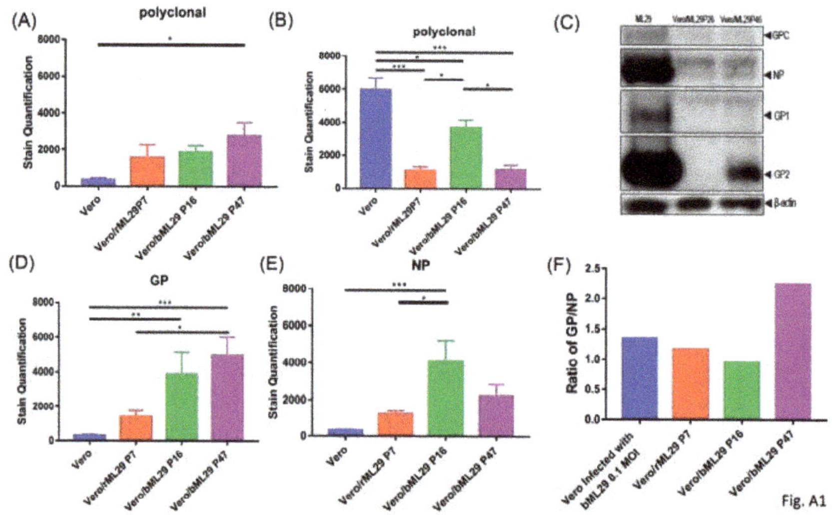

Figure A1. Quantification of immunofocus staining using polyclonal moneky-anti-ML29 on the indicated cell lines (**A**) without additional treatment, or (**B**) 3 days following infection with a 0.1 MOI of ML29. (**C**) Western blot of cell lysates from ML29, Vero/ML29P26, and Vero/ML29P46 detected with polyclonal monkey-anti-ML29 antibody. (**D–E**) Quantification of immunofocus staining using (**D**) polyclonal rabbit-anti-LASV-GP 1:400, or (**E**) mouse-anti-LASV/Jos-NP 1:100 antibodies. (**F**) The calculated ratio between staining quantified in (**D**) and (**E**). * $p < 0.05$, ** $p < 0.01$, *** $p < 0.001$.

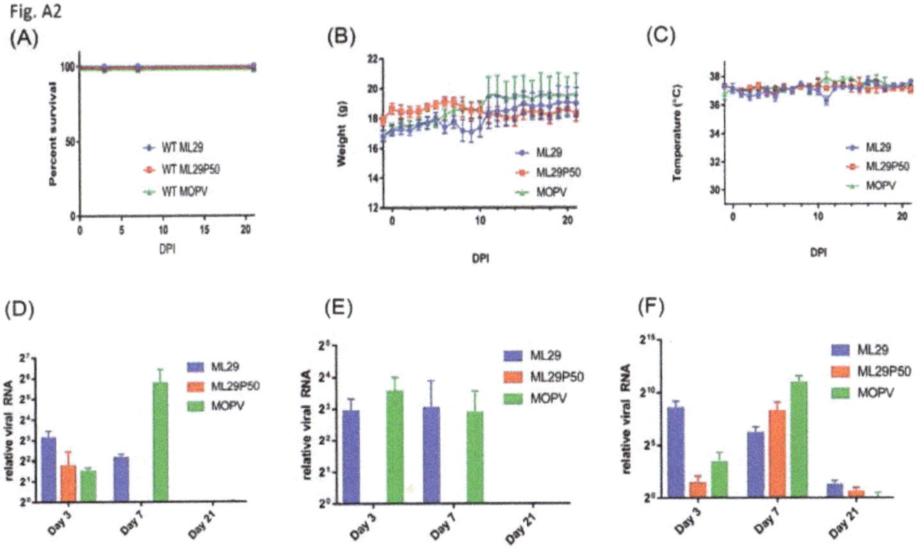

Figure A2. (**A**) Survival of wild-type 129S6 mice infected IP with 1×10^3 PFU of ML29, 1×10^3 PFU of MOPV, or a MOPV L gene qRT-PCR equivalent dose of supernatant from passage 50 Vero/ML29 cells. Daily (**B**) weight and (**C**) temperature of mice from (**A**). (**D–F**) Relative expression of MOPV L gene by qRT-PCR in the (**D**) liver, (**E**) spleen, and (**F**) kidney of wild-type 129S at the time points indicated post-infection.

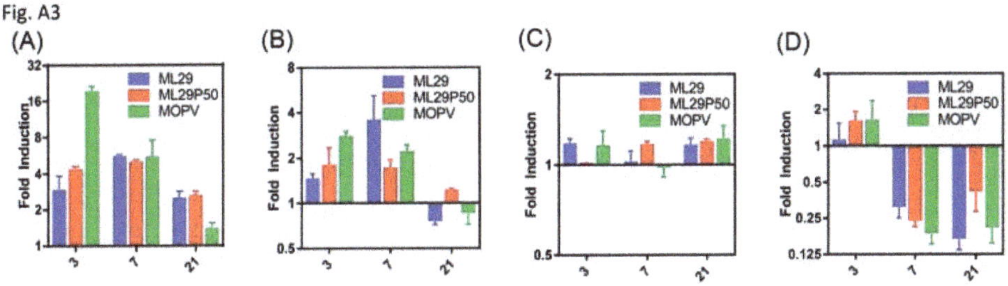

Figure A3. qRT-PCR analysis showing IL-6 expression in the (**A**) liver and (**B**) spleen, (**C**) TNF-α in the spleen, or (**D**) IL-1β expression in the spleen of wild-type 129S6 mice infected with the indicated viruses relative to mock infected at days 3, 7, and 21 post-infection.

Supplemental Materials and Methods

Quantification of immunofocus staining from high-quality images of scanned plates was performed using Adobe Photoshop to reduce background and threshold images followed by ImageJ counting of pixels. Statistical significance was tested with a one-way ANOVA using GraphPad Prism version 7.

For western blotting, a T-75 cell culture flask with a confluent monolayer of either Vero cells was infected with a 1 MOI of ML29 5 days prior, or Vero/ML29, was harvested in Tris-buffer containing 1.0% NP-40, protease inhibitors and 0.1% SDS. Protein content was standardized based on a pierce modified Lowry protein assay (ThermoFisher) denatured by boiling in Laemmli's buffer and run on a 10% acrylamide gel at 120 V for 1 h. The proteins were transferred to a nitrocellulose membrane, blocked with 5% milk, and detected with a 1:1000 dilution of polyclonal monkey-anti-ML29 antibody.

References

1. Frame, J.D.; Baldwin, J.M., Jr.; Gocke, D.J.; Troup, J.M. Lassa fever, a new virus disease of man from West Africa. I. Clinical description and pathological findings. *Am. J. Trop. Med. Hyg.* **1970**, *19*, 670–676. [CrossRef] [PubMed]
2. McCormick, J.B. Epidemiology and control of Lassa fever. *Curr. Top. Microbiol. Immunol.* **1987**, *134*, 69–78.
3. Fichet-Calvet, E.; Rogers, D.J. Risk Maps of Lassa Fever in West Africa. *PLoS Negl. Trop. Dis.* **2009**, *3*, e388. [CrossRef] [PubMed]
4. Richmond, J.K.; Baglole, D.J. Lassa fever: Epidemiology, clinical features, and social consequences. *BMJ* **2003**, *237*, 1271–1275. [CrossRef] [PubMed]
5. Sogoba, N.; Feldmann, H.; Safronetz, D. Lassa Fever in West Africa: Evidence for an Expanded Region of Endemicity. *Zoonoses Public Health* **2012**, *59*, 43–47. [CrossRef] [PubMed]
6. Bowen, M.; Rollin, P.E.; Ksiazek, T.G.; Hustad, H.L.; Buasch, D.G.; Demby, A.H.; Bjani, M.D.; Peters, C.J.; Nichol, S.T. Genetic diversity among Lassa virus strains. *J. Virol.* **2000**, *74*, 6992–7004. [CrossRef] [PubMed]
7. Andersen, K.G.; Shapiro, B.J.; Matranga, C.B.; Sealfon, R.; Lin, A.E.; Moses, L.M.; Floarin, O.A.; Goba, A.; Oida, I.; Ehiane, P.E.; et al. Clinical Sequencing Uncovers Origins and Evolution of Lassa Virus. *Cell* **2015**, *162*, 738–750. [CrossRef] [PubMed]
8. Emmerich, P.; Gunter, S.; Schmitz, H. Strain-specific antibody response to Lassa virus in the local population of West AFrica. *J. Clin. Virol.* **2008**, *42*, 40–44. [CrossRef] [PubMed]
9. Falzarano, D.; Feldmann, H. Vaccines for viral hemorrhagic fevers—Progress and shortcomings. *Curr. Opin. Virol.* **2013**, *3*, 1–9. [CrossRef] [PubMed]
10. Buba, M.I.; Dalhat, M.M.; Nguku, P.M.; Waziri, N.; Mohammad, J.O.; Bomoi, I.M.; Onyiah, A.P.; Balogun, M.S.; Bashorun, A.T.; et al. Mortality Among Confirmed Lassa Fever Cases During the 2015–2016 Outbreak in Nigeria. *Am. J. Public Health* **2017**, *108*, 262–264. [CrossRef] [PubMed]
11. Roberts, L. Nigeria hit by unprecedented Lassa fever outbreak. *Science* **2018**, *359*, 1201–1202. [CrossRef] [PubMed]
12. WHO. *Annual Review of Diseases Prioritized under the Research and Development Blueprint*; WHO: Geneva, Switzerland, 24–25 January 2017. Available online: http://www.who.int/blueprint/what/research-development/2017-Prioritization-Long-Report.pdf?ua=1 (accessed on 14 January 2019).
13. WHO. WHO Target Product Profile for Lassa Virus Vaccine. June 2017. Available online: http://www.who.int/blueprint/priority-diseases/key-action/LassaVirusVaccineTPP.PDF?ua=1 (accessed on 14 January 2019).
14. WHO. Lassa Fever. 2018. Available online: http://www.who.int/csr/don/20-april-2018-lassa-fever-nigeria/en/ (accessed on 14 January 2019).
15. Radoshitzky, S.R.; Bào, Y.; Buchmeier, M.J.; Charrel, R.N.; Clawson, A.N.; Clegg, C.S.; DeRisi, J.L.; Emonet, S.; Gonzalez, J.P.; Kuhn, J.H.; et al. Past, present, and future of arenavirus taxonomy. *Arch. Virol.* **2015**, *160*, 1851–1874. [CrossRef] [PubMed]
16. Wulff, H.; McIntosh, B.M.; Hamner, D.B.; Johnson, K.M. Isolation of an arenavirus closely related to Lassa virus from Mastomys natalensis in South-East Africa. *Bull. World Health Organ.* **1977**, *55*, 441–444. [PubMed]
17. Günther, S.; Hoofd, G.; Charrel, R.; Röser, C.; Becker-Ziaja, B.; Lloyd, G.; Sabuni, C.; Verhagen, R.; van der Groen, G.; Kennis, J.; Katakweba, A.; et al. Mopeia virus-related arenavirus in Natal multimammate mice, Morogoro, Tanzania. *Emerg. Infect. Dis.* **2009**, *15*, 2008–2010. [CrossRef] [PubMed]
18. Ishii, A.; Thomas, Y.; Moonga, L.; Nakamura, I.; Ohnuma, A.; Hang'ombe, B.; Takada, A.; Mweene, A.; Sawa, H. Novel arenavirus, Zambia. *Emerg. Infect. Dis.* **2011**, *17*, 1921–1924. [CrossRef]
19. Gryseels, S.; Rieger, T.; Oestereich, L.; Cuypers, B.; Borremans, B.; Makundi, R.; Leirs, H.; Günther, S.; Goüy de Bellocq, J. Gairo virus, a novel arenavirus of the widespread Mastomys natalensis: Genetically divergent, but ecologically similar to Lassa and Morogoro viruses. *Virology* **2015**, *476*, 249–256. [CrossRef]
20. Radoshitzky, S.R.; Kuhn, J.H.; Jahrling, P.B.; Bavari, S. Hemorrhagic Fever-Causing Mammarenaviruses. In *Medical Aspects of Biological Warfare*; Bozue, J., Cote, C.K., Glass, P.J., Eds.; Office of the Surgeon General: Fort Sam Houston, TX, USA, 2018; Chapter 21; pp. 517–545.
21. Riviere, Y.; Ahmed, R.; Southern, P.J.; Buchmeier, M.J.; Oldstone, M.B. Genetic mapping of lymphocytic choriomeningitis virus pathogenicity: Virulence in guinea pigs is associated with the L RNA segment. *J. Virol.* **1985**, *55*, 704–709.

22. Zhang, L.; Marriott, K.A.; Harnish, D.G.; Aronson, J.F. Reassortant analysis of guinea pig virulence of Pichinde virus variants. *Virology* **2001**, *290*, 30–38. [CrossRef]
23. Lukashevich, I.S.; Vasiuchkov, A.D.; Stel'makh, T.A.; Scheslenok, E.P.; Shabanov, A.G. The isolation and characteristics of reassortants between the Lassa and Mopeia arenaviruses. *Vopr. Virusol.* **1991**, *36*, 146–150.
24. Lukashevich, I.S. Generation of reassortants between African arenaviruses. *Virology* **1992**, *188*, 600–605. [CrossRef]
25. Lukashevich, I.S.; Patterson, J.; Carrion, R.; Moshkoff, D.; Ticer, A.; Zapata, J.; Brasky, K.; Geiger, R.; Hubbard, G.B.; Bryant, J.; et al. A Live Attenuated Vaccine for Lassa Fever Made by Reassortment of Lassa and Mopeia Viruses. *J. Virol.* **2005**, *79*, 13934–13942. [CrossRef]
26. Cohen, J. Unfilled Vials. *Science* **2016**, *351*, 16–19. [CrossRef] [PubMed]
27. Moshkoff, D.A.; Salvato, M.S.; Lukashevich, I.S. Molecular characterization of a reassortant virus derived from Lassa and Mopeia viruses. *Virus Genes* **2007**, *34*, 169–176. [CrossRef]
28. Lukashevich, I.; Carrion, R., Jr.; Salvato, M.S.; Mansfield, K.; Brasky, K.; Zapata, J.; Cairo, C.; Goicochea, M.; Hoosien, GE.; Ticer, A.; Bryant, J.; et al. Safety, immunogenicity, and efficacy of the ML29 reassortant vaccine for Lassa fever in small non-human primates. *Vaccine* **2008**, *26*, 5246–5254. [CrossRef] [PubMed]
29. Zapata, J.C.; Carrion, R., Jr.; Patterson, J.L.; Crasta, O.; Zhang, Y.; Mani, S.; Jett, M.; Poonia, B.; Djavani, M.; White, D.M.; et al. Transcriptome Analysis of Human Peripheral Blood Mononuclear Cells Exposed to Lassa Virus and to the Attenuated Mopeia/Lassa Reassortant 29 (ML29), a Vaccine Candidate. *PLoS Negl. Trop. Dis.* **2013**, *7*, e2406. [CrossRef]
30. Iwasaki, M.; Cubitt, B.; Jokinen, J.; Lukashevich, I.S.; de la Torre, J.C. Use of recombinant ML29 platform to generate polyvalent live-attenuated vaccines against lassa fever and other infectious diseases. In Proceedings of the 66th Annual Meeting of Japanese Society for Virology, Kyoto, Japan, 28–30 October 2018. Available online: http://www.c-linkage.co.jp/jsv66/data/pro_workshop_day1.pdf (accessed on 14 January 2019).
31. Lukashevich, I.S. The search for animal models for Lassa fever vaccine development. *Expert Rev. Vaccines* **2013**, *12*, 71–86. [CrossRef]
32. Fisher-Hoch, S.P.; Hutwagner, L.; Brown, B.; McCormick, J.B. Effective Vaccine for Lassa Fever. *J. Virol.* **2000**, *74*, 6777–6783. [CrossRef] [PubMed]
33. Prescott, J.B.; Marzi, A.; Safronetz, D.; Robertson, S.; Feldmann, H.; Best, S.M. Immunobiology of Ebola and Lassa virus infections. *Nat. Rev. Immunol.* **2017**, *17*, 195–207. [CrossRef] [PubMed]
34. Jahrling, P.B.; Smith, S.; Hesse, R.A.; Rhoderick, J.B. Pathogenesis of Lassa virus infection in guinea pigs. *Infect. Immunity* **1982**, *37*, 771–778.
35. Peters, C.; Jahrling, P.B.; Lui, C.T.; Kenyon, R.H.; McKee, K.T., Jr.; Barrera Oro, J.G. Experimental studies of arenaviral hemorrhagic fevers. *Curr. Top. Microbiol. Immunol.* **1987**, *134*, 5–68.
36. Bell, T.M.; Shaia, C.I.; Bearss, J.J.; Mattix, M.E.; Koistinen, K.A.; Honnold, S.P.; Zeng, X.; Blancett, C.D.; Donnelly, G.C.; Shamblin, J.D.; et al. Temporal Progression of Lesions in Guinea Pigs Infected with Lassa Virus. *Vet. Pathol.* **2017**, *54*, 549–562. [CrossRef] [PubMed]
37. Jahrling, P.B.; Frame, J.D.; Smith, S.B.; Monson, M.H. Endemic Lassa fever in Liberia. III. Characterization of Lassa virus isolates. *Trans. R. Soc. Trop. Med. Hyg.* **1985**, *79*, 374–379. [CrossRef]
38. Morrison, H.; Bauer, S.P.; Lange, J.V.; Esposito, J.J.; McCormick, J.B.; Auperin, D.D. Protection of guinea pigs from Lassa fever by vaccinia virus recombinants expressing the nucleoprotein or the envelope glycoproteins of Lassa virus. *Virology* **1989**, *171*, 179–188. [CrossRef]
39. Pushko, P.; Geisbert, J.; Parker, M.; Jarling, P.; Smith, J. Individual and bivalent vaccines based on alphavirus replicons protect guinea pigs against infection with Lassa and Ebola viruses. *J. Virol.* **2001**, *75*, 11677–11685. [CrossRef] [PubMed]
40. Golden, J.W.; Hammerbeck, C.D.; Mucker, E.M.; Brocato, R.L. Animal Models for the Study of Rodent-Borne Hemorrhagic Fever Viruses: Arenaviruses and Hantaviruses. *BioMed Res. Int.* **2015**, *2015*, 793257. [CrossRef] [PubMed]
41. Yun, N.E.; Seregin, A.V.; Walker, D.H.; Popov, V.L.; Walker, A.G.; Smith, J.N.; Miller, M.; de la Torre, J.C.; Smith, J.K.; Borisevich, V.; et al. Mice lacking functional STAT1 are highly susceptable to lethal infection with Lassa virus. *J. Virol.* **2013**, *87*, 10908–10911. [CrossRef] [PubMed]
42. Yun, N.E.; Ronca, S.; Tamura, A.; Koma, T.; Seregin, A.V.; Dineley, K.T.; Miller, M.; Cook, R.; Shimizu, N.; Walker, A.G.; et al. Animal Model of Sensorineural Hearing Loss Associated with Lassa Virus Infection. *J. Virol.* **2016**, *90*, 2920–2927. [CrossRef]

43. López, C.B. Defective Viral Genomes: Critical Danger Signals of Viral Infections. *J. Virol.* **2014**, *88*, 8720–8723. [CrossRef]
44. Rezelj, V.V.; Levi, L.I.; Vignuzzi, M. The defective component of viral populations. *Curr. Opin. Virol.* **2018**, *33*, 74–80. [CrossRef]
45. Baltes, A.; Akpinar, F.; Inankur, B.; Yin, J. Inhibition of infection spread by co-transmitted defective interfering particles. *PLoS ONE* **2017**, *12*, e0184029. [CrossRef]
46. McLaren, L.; Holland, J. Defective interfering particles from poliovirus vaccine and vaccine reference strains. *Virology* **1974**, *60*, 579–583. [CrossRef]
47. Frensing, T. Defective interfering viruses and their impact on vaccines and viral vectors. *Biotechnol. J.* **2015**, *10*, 681–689. [CrossRef] [PubMed]
48. Gould, P.S.; Easton, A.J.; Dimmock, N.J. Live Attenuated Influenza Vaccine contains Substantial and Unexpected Amounts of Defective Viral Genomic RNA. *Viruses* **2017**, *9*, 269. [CrossRef] [PubMed]
49. Calain, P.; Roux, L. Generation of measles virus defective interfering particles and their presence in a preparation of attenuated live-virus vaccine. *J. Virol.* **1988**, *62*, 2859–2866. [PubMed]
50. Whistler, T.; Bellini, W.J.; Rota, P.A. Generation of Defective Interfering Particles by Two Vaccine Strains of Measles Virus. *Virology* **1996**, *220*, 480–484. [CrossRef] [PubMed]
51. Ho, T.H.; Kew, C.; Lui, P.Y.; Chan, C.P.; Satoh, T.; Akira, S.; Jin, D.Y.; Kok, K.H. PACT- and RIG-I-Dependent Activation of Type I Interferon Production by a Defective Interfering RNA Derived from Measles Virus Vaccine. *J. Virol.* **2016**, *90*, 1557–1568. [CrossRef] [PubMed]
52. Dutko, F.J.; Pfau, C.J. Arenavirus Defective Interfering Particles Mask the Cell-Killing Potential of Standard Virus. *J. Gen. Virol.* **1978**, *38*, 195–208. [CrossRef]
53. Popescu, M.; Schaefer, H.; Lehmann-Grube, F. Homologous interference of lymphocytic choriomeningitis virus: Detection and measurement of interference focus-forming units. *J. Virol.* **1976**, *20*, 1–8.
54. Welsh, R.M.; Connell, C.M.; Pfau, C.J. Properties of Defective Lymphocytic Choriomeningitis Virus. *J. Gen. Virol.* **1972**, *17*, 355–359. [CrossRef]
55. Welsh, R.M.; Burner, P.A.; Holland, J.J.; Oldstone, M.B.; Thompson, H.A.; Villarreal, L.P. A comparison of biochemical and biological properties of standard and defective lymphocytic choriomeningitis virus. *Bull. World Health Organ.* **1975**, *52*, 403–408.
56. Welsh, R.; Lampert, P.W.; Oldstone, M.B. Prevention of virus-induced cerebellar diseases by defective-interfering lymphocytic choriomeningitis virus. *J. Infect. Dis.* **1977**, *136*, 391–399. [CrossRef] [PubMed]
57. Welsh, R.; Oldstone, M.B.A. Inhibition of immunologic injury of cultered cells infected with lymphocytic choriomeningitis virus: Role of defective interfering virus in regulating viral antigen expression. *J. Exp. Med.* **1977**, *145*, 1449–1468. [CrossRef] [PubMed]
58. Popescu, M.; Lehmann-Grube, F. Defective interfering particles in mice infected with lymphocytic choriomeningitis virus. *Virology* **1977**, *77*, 78–83. [CrossRef]
59. Lukashevich, I.S.; Mar'iankova, R.F.; Fidarov, F.M. Acute and chronic Lassa virus infection of Vero cells. *Vopr. Virusol.* **1981**, *4*, 452–456.
60. Lukashevich, I.S.; Mar'iankova, R.F.; Lemeshko, N.N. Autointerfering activity of Lassa virus. *Vopr. Virusol.* **1983**, *1*, 96–101.
61. Lukashevich, I.S.; Trofimov, N.M.; Golibev, V.P.; Maryankova, R.F. Sedimentation analysis of the RNAs isolated from interfering particles of Lassa and Machupo viruses. *Acta Virol.* **1985**, *29*, 455–460. [PubMed]
62. Goicochea, M.A.; Zapata, J.C.; Bryant, J.; Davis, H.; Salvato, M.S.; Lukashevich, I.S. Evaluation of Lassa virus vaccine immunogenicity in a CBA/J-ML29 mouse model. *Vaccine* **2012**, *30*, 1445–1452. [CrossRef]
63. Wang, M.; Jokinen, J.; Tretyakova, I.; Pushko, P.; Lukashevich, I.S. Alphavirus vector-based replicon particles expressing multivalent cross-protective Lassa virus glycoproteins. *Vaccine* **2018**, *36*, 683–690. [CrossRef] [PubMed]
64. Kiley, M.P.; Swanepoel, R.; Mitchell, S.W.; Lange, J.V.; Gonzalez, J.P.; McCormick, J.B. Serological and biological evidence that Lassa-complex arenaviruses are widely distributed in Africa. *Med. Microbiol. Immunol.* **1986**, *175*, 161–163. [CrossRef] [PubMed]
65. Kiley, M.P.; Lange, J.V.; Johnson, K.M. Protection of rhesus monkeys from Lassa virus by immunisation with closely related Arenavirus. *Lancet* **1979**, *2*, 738. [CrossRef]

66. Safronetz, D.; Strong, J.E.; Feldmann, F.; Haddock, E.; Sogoba, N.; Brining, D.; Geisbert, T.W.; Scott, D.P.; Feldmann, H. A Recently Isolated Lassa Virus from Mali Demonstrates Atypical Clinical Disease Manifestations and Decreased Virulence in Cynomolgus Macaques. *J. Infect. Dis.* **2013**, *207*, 1316–1327. [CrossRef] [PubMed]
67. Russier, M.; Pannetier, D.; Baize, S. Immune Responses and Lassa Virus Infection. *Viruses* **2012**, *4*, 2766–2785. [CrossRef] [PubMed]
68. Hallam, H.J.; Hallman, S.; Rodriguez, S.E.; Barrett, A.D.T.; Beasley, D.W.C.; Chau, A.; Ksiazek, T.G.; Milligan, G.N.; Sathiyamoorthy, V.; Reece, L.M. Baseline mapping of Lassa fever virology, epidemiology and vaccine research and development. *NPJ Vaccines* **2018**, *3*, 11. [CrossRef] [PubMed]
69. McElroy, A.K.; Akondy, R.S.; Harmon, J.R.; Ellebedy, A.H.; Cannon, D.; Klena, J.D.; Sidney, J.; Sette, A.; Mehta, A.K.; Kraft, C.S. A Case of Human Lassa Virus Infection with Robust Acute T-Cell Activation and Long-Term Virus-Specific T-Cell Responses. *J. Infect. Dis.* **2017**, *215*, 1862–1872. [CrossRef] [PubMed]
70. Huang, A.S.; Baltimore, D. Defective interfering particles of animal viruses. *Comput. Virol.* **1977**, *10*, 73–116.
71. Huang, A.S. Defective Interfering Viruses. *Annu. Rev. Microbiol.* **1973**, *27*, 101–118. [CrossRef] [PubMed]
72. Barrett, A.D.; Dimmock, N.J. Defective interfering viruses and infections of animals. *Curr. Top. Microbiol. Immunol.* **1986**, *128*, 55–84.
73. Perrault, J. Origin and replication of defective interfering particles. *Curr. Top. Microbiol. Immunol.* **1981**, *93*, 151–207.
74. Roux, L.; Simon, A.E.; Holland, J.J. Effects of defective interfering viruses on virus replication and pathogenesis in vitro and in vivo. *Adv. Virus Res.* **1991**, *40*, 181–211.
75. Lukashevich, I.S.; Salvato, M.S. Lassa Virus Genome. *Curr. Genet.* **2006**, *7*, 351–379. [CrossRef]
76. Lukashevich, I.S.; Vela, E.M. Pathogenesis of Lasa virus infection in experimentl animals. In *Molecular Pathogenesis of Viral Hemorrhagic Fevers*; Vela, E.M., Ed.; Transworld Research Network: Kerala, India, 2010; pp. 101–142.
77. Peralta, L.M.; Bruns, M.; Lehmann-Grube, F. Biochemical composition of lymphocytic choriomeningitis virus interfering particles. *J. Gen. Virol.* **1981**, *55*, 475–479. [CrossRef] [PubMed]
78. Meyer, B.; Southern, P. A novel type of defective viral genome suggests a unique strategy to establish and maintain persistent lymphocytic choriomeningitis virus infections. *J. Virol.* **1997**, *71*, 6757–6764. [PubMed]
79. Cornu, T.I.; Feldmann, H.; de la Torre, J.C. Cells Expressing the RING Finger Z Protein Are Resistant to Arenavirus Infection. *J. Virol.* **2004**, *78*, 2979–2983. [CrossRef] [PubMed]
80. Zaza, A.D.; Herbreteau, C.H.; Peyrefitte, C.N.; Emonet, S.F. Mammarenaviruses deleted from their Z gene are replicative and produce an infectious progeny in BHK-21 cells. *Virology* **2018**, *518*, 34–44. [CrossRef] [PubMed]
81. Xing, J.; Ly, H.; Liang, Y. The Z Proteins of Pathogenic but Not Nonpathogenic Arenaviruses Inhibit RIG-i-Like Receptor-Dependent Interferon Production. *J. Virol.* **2015**, *89*, 944–2955. [CrossRef] [PubMed]
82. Sun, Y.; Jain, D.; Koziol-White, C.J.; Genoyer, E.; Gilbert, M.; Tapia, K.; Panettieri, R.A., Jr.; Hodinka, R.L.; López, C.B. Immunostimulatory Defective Viral Genomes from Respiratory Syncytial Virus Promote a Strong Innate Antiviral Response during Infection in Mice and Humans. *PLoS Pathog.* **2015**, *11*, e1005122. [CrossRef] [PubMed]
83. Lukashevich, I.S.; Pushko, P. Vaccine platforms to control Lassa fever. *Expert Rev. Vaccines* **2016**, *15*, 1135–1150. [CrossRef] [PubMed]
84. Carrion, R., Jr.; Patterson, J.L.; Johnson, C.; Gonzales, M.; Moreira, C.R.; Ticer, A.; Brasky, K.; Hubbard, G.B.; Moshkoff, D.; Zapata, J.; et al. A ML29 reassortant virus protects guinea pigs against a distantly related Nigerian strain of Lassa virus and can provide sterilizing immunity. *Vaccine* **2007**, *25*, 4093–4102. [CrossRef] [PubMed]
85. Zapata, J.; Medina-Moreno, S.; Guzmán-Cardozo, C.; Salvato, M.S. Improving the Breadth of the Host's Immune Response to Lassa Virus. *Pathogens* **2018**, *7*, 84. [CrossRef]

pathogens

MDPI

Article

A Single Dose of Modified Vaccinia Ankara Expressing Lassa Virus-like Particles Protects Mice from Lethal Intra-cerebral Virus Challenge

Maria S. Salvato [1,†], Arban Domi [2,†], Camila Guzmán-Cardozo [1], Sandra Medina-Moreno [1], Juan Carlos Zapata [1], Haoting Hsu [1], Nathanael McCurley [3], Rahul Basu [4], Mary Hauser [2], Michael Hellerstein [2] and Farshad Guirakhoo [2,*]

1 Institute of Human Virology, University of Maryland, Baltimore, MD 21201, USA
2 GeoVax, Inc., Smyrna, GA 30080, USA
3 Office of Technology Licensing and Commercialization, Georgia State University, Atlanta, GA 30303, USA
4 Department of Biology, Georgia State University, Atlanta, GA 30302, USA
* Correspondence: fguirakhoo@geovax.com
† Contributed equally to this work.

Received: 17 July 2019; Accepted: 25 August 2019; Published: 28 August 2019

Abstract: Lassa fever surpasses Ebola, Marburg, and all other hemorrhagic fevers except Dengue in its public health impact. Caused by Lassa virus (LASV), the disease is a scourge on populations in endemic areas of West Africa, where reported incidence is higher. Here, we report construction, characterization, and preclinical efficacy of a novel recombinant vaccine candidate GEO-LM01. Constructed in the Modified Vaccinia Ankara (MVA) vector, GEO-LM01 expresses the glycoprotein precursor (GPC) and zinc-binding matrix protein (Z) from the prototype Josiah strain lineage IV. When expressed together, GP and Z form Virus-Like Particles (VLPs) in cell culture. Immunogenicity and efficacy of GEO-LM01 was tested in a mouse challenge model. A single intramuscular dose of GEO-LM01 protected 100% of CBA/J mice challenged with a lethal dose of ML29, a Mopeia/Lassa reassortant virus, delivered directly into the brain. In contrast, all control animals died within one week. The vaccine induced low levels of antibodies but Lassa-specific $CD4^+$ and $CD8^+$ T cell responses. This is the first report showing that a single dose of a replication-deficient MVA vector can confer full protection against a lethal challenge with ML29 virus.

Keywords: Lassa vaccine; replication-deficient MVA vector; VLP formation; single-dose efficacy; cell-mediated immunity

1. Introduction

Lassa fever (LF), a zoonotic disease caused by Lassa virus (LASV), can lead to acute hemorrhagic fever with a case fatality rate (CFR) of up to 50% [1]. The estimated annual incidence of LF across West African countries including Ghana, Guinea, Mali, Benin, Liberia, Sierra Leone, Togo, and Nigeria has been reported as high as 300,000 infections and 5000–10,000 deaths, but these figures are most likely underestimates due to inadequate diagnosis and surveillance [2–5]. Based on prospective studies performed in Guinea, Sierra Leone, Liberia, and Nigeria, it was estimated that 59 million people are at risk of LASV infections, with as many as 67,000 deaths per year [6]. The 2018 outbreak in Nigeria resulted in 3498 suspected cases in 22 states and 171 deaths with a CFR of 27% based on confirmed cases [7]. The fact that a virus that was first discovered in 1969 in Lassa village in Nigeria is still capable of causing outbreaks in the same geographical regions indicates challenges in eradicating its animal reservoir.

The main animal reservoir of LASV is the multimammate rat (*Mastomys natalensis*), which is common in West Africa, but the potential transmission of LASV to new rodent hosts could have serious implications for its spread beyond West Africa [8]. LASV is mainly transmitted to humans by consumption of contaminated food, by contact with rodent urine and droppings, or by inhalation of virus particles from the excreta of infected animals; it can also be transmitted from human to human through nosocomial infections [9]. Most LASV infections are asymptomatic or cause only mild symptoms, but some infections lead to multi-organ failure, fever, and, on occasion, hemorrhage and death [10,11].

LASV is a member of the family *Arenaviridae* and genus *Mammarenavirus*, which includes Old World and New World arenaviruses [12,13]. Furthermore, LASV strains are classified into four lineages, I–IV (with a newly proposed fifth lineage from Cote d'lvoire and Mali) based on their genetic variations [12,13]. The LASV genome is composed of two ambisense RNA segments. The large (L) segment of 7.2 kb in length encodes the viral RNA-dependent RNA polymerase protein and the zinc finger (Z) protein, a multifunctional matrix protein [14,15]. The small (S) segment of 3.4 kb in length encodes the nucleoprotein (NP) and glycoprotein precursor (GPC). GPC is cleaved post-translationally to form a trimer of hetero-trimers, each consisting of a receptor binding protein (GP1), a fusion protein (GP2) and a stable signal peptide (SSP) [16,17]. GPC sequences, shown previously to be required for full protection, have been used as the protective antigen in the construction of a large number of vaccine candidates delivered by various platforms. Some of these candidates have undergone preclinical evaluations in mice, guinea pigs, and non-human primates (NHP) [12], and a DNA vaccine has entered clinical trials [18].

Here, we describe the construction, characterization and efficacy of a Lassa vaccine candidate that generates virus-like particles (VLPs) by expression of Lassa GPC and Z proteins from our Modified Vaccinia Ankara (MVA) vector. It has been previously demonstrated that co-expression of Z and GP proteins leads to the formation of VLPs [19]. A murine model was chosen initially to establish dose and route of vaccination and whether our constructs could elicit any protective immunity. In this model, ML29, an attenuated Mopeia -Lassa (MOP/LAS) reassortant, is delivered into the brain and primarily infects brain capillary endothelial and glial cells that present LASV antigens, triggering an influx of lymphocytes 5–6 days later. The infiltrating cells contribute to encephalitis that is lethal unless the mice had been previously vaccinated against LASV (Djavani and Salvato, unpublished). The intra-cerebral (IC) delivery we used was not "natural", since it models brain infections that are rare in LF, but it allows a rapid and simple read-out for whether or not we elicited a protective immunity. Here, we show that a single dose of the vaccine conferred full protection against a lethal challenge dose of the ML29 virus delivered IC.

2. Results

2.1. Vaccine Characterization

The recombinant GEO-LM01 was constructed by inserting sequences from the well-characterized LASV prototype strain Josiah from lineage IV into MVA. The Josiah strain is extensively used for vaccine development, since it has shown protection against homologous and heterologous challenges [20]. The GPC protein of Josiah, the major protective antigen, has 93.1%, 93.5, and 94.5% homologies with lineage I, II, and III, respectively [12]. GEO-LM01 is designed to co-express GPC and the LASV matrix protein Z (Figure 1a,b). Expression of GPC and Z lead to the formation of VLPs in the cells of the inoculated host as well as promoting their release from GEO-LM01-infected cells. GEO-LM01 is replication-competent in avian cells (producing both infectious progeny and expressed antigens) but is replication-deficient in mammalian cells (producing antigens in the form of VLPs but not infectious progeny) (Figure 1c) due to six deletions in the MVA genome which together resulted in high attenuation and mammalian cell host restriction [21]. The assembly of VLPs from proteins expressed by GEO-LM01 was verified by electron microscopy, demonstrating active release of VLPs from DF1 cells, a chicken fibroblast cell line (Figure 2a). The entire population of GEO-LM01 virions retains both GPC and Z transgenes as demonstrated by immunostaining (Figure 2b). Similar plaque numbers at each dilution in the GPC and Z wells showed that both transgenes are equally retained. Expression of both transgenes and cleavage of GPC into GP1 and GP2 subunits was further demonstrated in western blots (WB) using cell lysates and supernatants (released VLPs) of GEO-LM01 infected DF1 cells (Figure 2c,d).

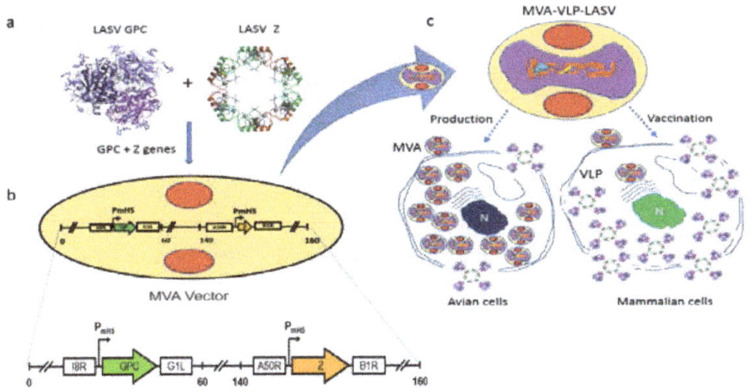

Figure 1. Construction of GEO-LM01 vaccine candidate. A Cartoon showing the vector design. (**a**,**b**) The Lassa virus (LASV) sequence for glycoprotein precursor (GPC) was inserted between the I8R and G1L genes and the Z sequence was inserted between the A50R and B1R genes. P_{mH5}, modified H5 promoter. Numbers are coordinates in the Modified Vaccinia Ankara (MVA) genome. (**c**) Similar to all MVA-derived vaccine viruses, GEO-LM01 is replication-competent in avian cells, used for propagation of the vaccine but replication-deficient in mammalian cells that are used for vaccination purposes. Image of the LASV GPC protein structure is courtesy of Dr. Erica O. Saphire, The Scripps Research Institute. The image of LASV Z structure is from RCSB PDB (www.rcsb.org) ID 5I72 [22].

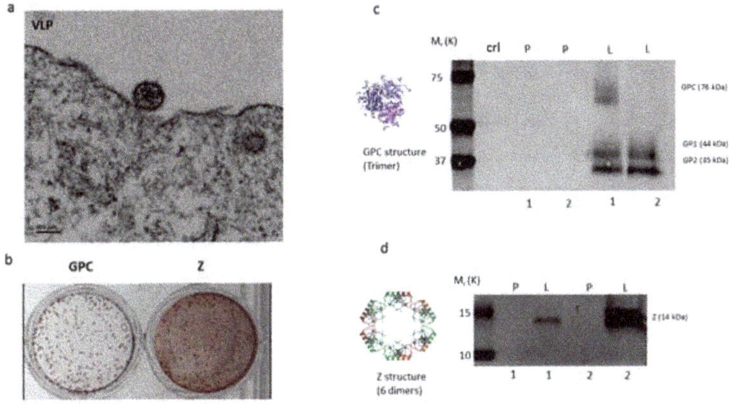

Figure 2. Electron microscopy, Immunocytochemistry and Western blot of GEO-LM01 vaccine candidate. (**a**) Electron micrograph of virus-like particles (VLP) formed in cells infected with GEO-LM01. (**b**) Immunocytochemistry on infected duplicates of cell monolayers stained with GPC- (left) or Z- (right) specific antibodies. Western blots verified expression of LASV GP (**c**) and Z (**d**) proteins in cultured cells. DF1 cell lysates contained both the unprocessed GPC and the processed subunits GP1 and GP2, whereas the DF1 supernatants contained only the processed GP1 and GP2 subunits. P, Parental (empty) MVA; L, GEO-LM01; 1, cell lysate; 2, supernatant. A loading control lane (**crl lane c**) served as another negative control. The two GP bands correspond to LASV GP1 and GP2 with the molecular weights of 44kD and 35kD, respectively.

2.2. *Vaccine Efficacy Testing in a ML29 Mouse Challenge Model*

Immunogenicity and efficacy testing of GEO-LM01 was performed in a mouse model that uses ML29 virus for lethal challenge (Figure 3). In this model, young immune-competent CBA/J mice are vaccinated once and challenged 2 weeks later. Animals are monitored for weight loss, morbidity, and mortality. Blood and spleens from three mice were collected on day 11 prior to challenge for determination of vaccine-elicited antibody and T cell responses, respectively.

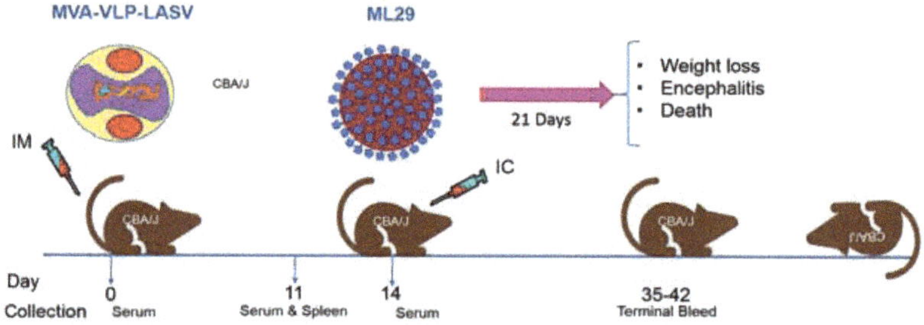

Figure 3. ML29 challenge model; schedule of vaccination, sample collections and intracerebral (IC) challenge. CBA/J mice are vaccinated with a single dose of GEO-LM01 (MVA-VLP-LASV) (1×10^7 $TCID_{50}$ in 100 μL volume) by the intramuscular (IM) route. Three mice are sacrificed on day 11, sera and spleens were collected for assessment of antibody and T cell responses. The remaining mice are challenged on day 14 by the IC route with 1000 plaque forming units (PFU) of ML29 virus. After challenge, mice are observed for weight loss, signs of encephalitis and death.

ML29 is a reassortant virus encoding the GPC and NP proteins of LASV (Josiah strain) and the L and Z proteins of MOPV virus [23]. The virus is uniformly lethal when administered by IC inoculation into immunocompetent CBA/J mice; however, when administered by intraperitoneal (IP) inoculation, ML29 elicits a strong immune response that protects CBA/J mice from death upon subsequent IC challenge [24]. To determine the best route of immunization, 4–6 week-old CBA/J mice were immunized with 10^7 $TCID_{50}$ of GEO-LM01 by IP, IM, or SC inoculation. Additionally, two groups of mice (n = 6) were injected IP with ML29 virus (1000 PFU) or saline, and served as positive and negative controls, respectively. On day 14, all mice were challenged by IC inoculation with ML29 virus and monitored for weight change, morbidity, and mortality. Mice immunized with ML29 virus (IP) (positive control) or with GEO-LM01 (IM) were 100% protected from lethal challenge and gained weight throughout the study (Figure 4a), whereas mice administered saline alone all died on day 7 or 8 after lethal challenge (Figure 4b). Some mice in the vaccinated groups exhibited minor weight loss after challenge, but they all regained weight and remained healthy (no ataxia or ruffled fur) until the end of the study. Mice immunized with GEO-LM01 by SC and IP administration showed less robust immunity to lethal challenge, as seen in the more appreciable weight loss in these groups as well as the death of one animal in each group (one animal in the SC group died early on day 2 post challenge, most likely due to problems with inoculation rather than virus growth; it was excluded from survival analysis). A second experiment to measure immunogenicity and efficacy was initiated in the same model system, in this instance examining only two conditions: Immunization with GEO-LM01 by IM inoculation (n = 10) and mock immunization with saline (n = 8) (Figure 4c). Spleens were harvested from immunized animals (n = 3) and saline-inoculated animals (n = 3) on day 11 after a single administration of the vaccine.

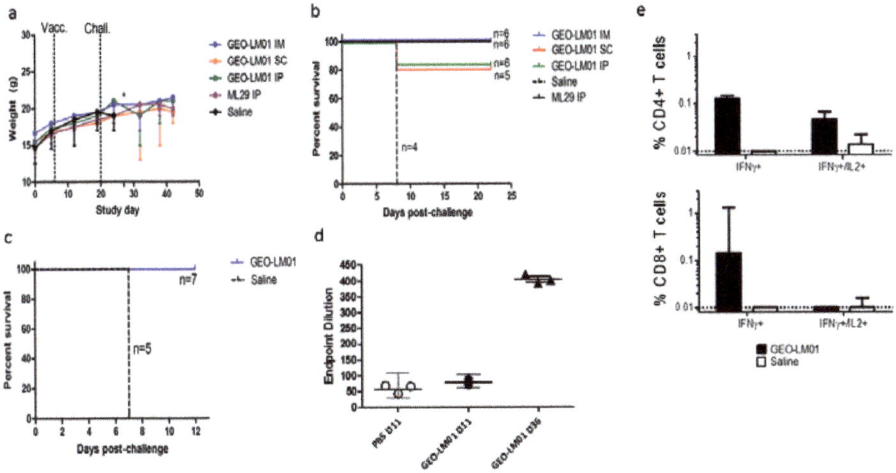

Figure 4. Efficacy and immunogenicity of GEO-LM01. Weight loss (**a**) and survival curves (**b**) following immunization by various routes then challenged with IC with ML29 virus 14 days later. * demonstrates death of control animals. (**c**) Survival curves of animals vaccinated by IM route only. (**d**) ML29-specific Ab titers from immunized on days 11 and 36 (22 days after challenge) and mock-immunized mice on day 11 as determined by ELISA. (**e**) Percentage of antigen-specific CD4+ and CD8+ T cells expressing IFNγ and IL2 in response to LASV GP peptides from GEO-LM01 or saline immunized animals were assessed by flow cytometry. These data demonstrate considerable differences between immunization groups but are not statistically significant.

Antigen-specific T cell responses were measured by Intracellular Cytokine Staining (ICS) for IFNγ and IL2 production by stimulating with peptides derived from immuno-dominant epitopes (IDE) present in GP1 and GP2 subunits [24–26]. IFNγ expression was evident in both CD4+ and CD8+ T cells of immunized but not mock immunized mice (Figure 4e). Some CD4+ T cells were also shown to be double positive for IFNγ and IL2, suggesting an expanding population. The remaining seven vaccinated and five control animals were challenged on day 14 as in the first experiment. All vaccinated animals survived the challenge, whereas all controls died by day 7 (Figure 4c) confirming the 100% single-dose efficacy of GEO-LM01 observed in the previous study. Four of the surviving GEO-LM01-vaccinated mice were housed for an additional year to see if they would be able to survive a second challenge long after the initial challenge. All four survived their second IC challenge (Table 1). A true test of durable immunity would not use mice surviving lethal challenge because the ML29 challenge itself may boost vaccine immunity; a better test would be to vaccinate mice and leave them unchallenged for a year to see whether or not the single vaccination could confer durable year-long protection.

Table 1. Surviving mice from Experiment 2 were re-challenged [1] one year later.

Experimental Mice	Number of Mice	Survivors after 2nd Challenge
Survivors of 1st challenge	4	4
Control mice (naïve adult CBA/J)	4	0

[1] All mice were challenged with a lethal dose of ML29 to see if the original vaccinated survivors could survive a second lethal challenge a year later. The naïve mice served as negative controls.

We additionally assayed for the presence of binding antibody (bAb) to GPC in the serum of the immunized mice. Despite the excellent protection from death afforded by GEO-LM01, we found no statistically significant level of bAb above background, we found low bAb at the early sampling days

11–14 post vaccination (Figure 4d). Similar results were observed previously with an ML29 vaccine that conferred protection from lethal challenge but yielded a minimal amount of bAb and neutralizing antibody (nAb) [24]. Substantial bAb were found in mice 36d after vaccination (Figure 4d) but these had been ML29 challenged, which could serve to boost the response to LASV antigens. We did not look for neutralizing antibodies.

3. Discussion

LF has a greater human impact than any other hemorrhagic fever, with the exception of Dengue fever [6]. Despite the severe impact of LF on populations in West Africa, no effective and practical medical countermeasure is available [18]. The one available treatment is the antiviral drug ribavirin, which is effective only if given within six days after infection [18]. A vaccine against LASV would be an ideal solution to the problem of LF, especially given the growing threat of outbreaks due to globalization and increased travel [27]. Several groups have developed vaccine candidates that have shown activity against LASV in animal models [20,23], but only one has progressed to the clinic [18]. Although a multi-dose immunization regiment is logistically feasible for medical providers and military personnel, a single dose vaccine is critical for epidemic response and is preferable and much more practical in under-resourced endemic areas. LF has been listed in the WHO R&D Blueprint among the 10 diseases and pathogens to prioritize for research and development in public health emergency contexts [28]. These diseases are identified as those that pose a public health risk because of their epidemic potential and for which there are insufficient countermeasures. For this reason, CEPI (Coalition for Epidemic Preparedness Innovations), founded to address the threat of epidemic diseases, has set aside a major portion of its $1 billion budget for the development of vaccines against LF [29].

GEO-LM01 provides a unique combination of advantages required for visitors or residents of LASV endemic countries. The potential for GEO-LM01 to protect after a single dose is favorable for travelers and military personnel who require a rapid onset of immunity (ideally ~<2 weeks post vaccination) as well as for epidemic/endemic vaccinations (due to the urgency of epidemic response and the complexity of locating vaccinated subjects in rural villages to administer a second dose for routine vaccination campaigns).

The GEO-LM01 reported here is designed to produce secreted as well as cell-associated LASV proteins in VLP (GPC+Z) formations in vaccinated subjects. This vaccine thereby provides two sources of viral antigens that mimic a natural viral infection promoting predominantly a balanced T cell response, which is critical for protection against LASV infection [30,31].

In our murine model, antibody responses occur too late to protect from an acute viral infection. We assessed binding antibodies in ML29-coated ELISA plates that are able to detect both the GP and Z components of VLP. Unfortunately, half of the Z protein is comprised of a RING structure that is common to many ligases and transcription factors in the normal cell, so it cross-reacts with many other proteins. In a recent publication [30], we posit that the value of the Z in VLP vectors is mostly to boost immunity by forming a 3-D structure with GP since conformational antigens are more immunogenic than linear antigens (boosting both CD4 and B cell responses).

As a vaccine candidate, GEO-LM01 has a unique combination of advantages that could potentially meet the preferred Target Product Profiles (TPP) of a LASV vaccine set by the WHO for both non-emergency (Preventive Use) and emergency settings (Reactive/Outbreak use) [28]. These include the immunological advantages of a live but safe (replication-deficient) vector that produces conformationally relevant VLPs; inclusion of multiple genes of LASV (GPC and Z) for induction of potentially broad immunity; the ability to immunize sequentially or concurrently with other MVA-vectored vaccines without generating any vector immunity [32] (potentially even combining GEO-LM01 with other hemorrhagic fever vaccines in a multivalent formulation); the likelihood of single-dose protection, as demonstrated with MVA-VLP-EBOV and MVA-Zika vaccines candidates [32,33] with the durability of the immune response attributed to MVA-vectored vaccines; and a temperature stable, simple, adjuvant-free presentation.

Considering the high prevalence of HIV in some LASV endemic areas of Sub-Saharan Africa (up to 68% in some populations) [34], an LASV vaccine must be safe and effective in immunocompromised populations [35]. Safety for the parental MVA vector was shown in more than 120,000 subjects in Europe, including immunocompromised individuals, during the initial development of MVA as a "safer smallpox vaccine" [36,37]. Furthermore, MVA has shown no reproductive toxicity in studies in pregnant rabbits or rats [38], and was used as a vector for malaria, influenza, and tuberculosis vaccines as well for cancer therapies in over 100 clinical trials since 1999 [32,33,39]. Our MVA-VLP HIV vaccine has demonstrated outstanding safety in clinical trials involving 500 humans [40,41], including immunocompromised individuals as well as HIV patients [40–42].

In this paper, we demonstrated that a single dose of GEO-LM01 confered full protection against the challenge virus ML29, which was directly inoculated into the brain. ML29 virus itself confers protection by the peripheral route, but its classification as a Risk group 3 (BSL3) agent creates major challenges for manufacturing in the US; in Europe it is considered Risk group 2 (BSL2). Similarly, commercial yellow fever (YF) vaccines (strains 17D and 17DD), approved more than half a century ago, are lethal for immunocompetent mice when inoculated by the IC route but can confer protection when administered by peripheral routes [43]. These strains are used as challenge viruses for the evaluation of new vaccines against YF virus. Our future work will continue in Hartley guinea pigs and NHP models (e.g., in cynomolgous macaques where signs of LASV infection mirror human disease) with live LASV under high laboratory containment, that is, Animal BSL4 (ABSL4) where the challenge virus is fully lethal by the parenteral route.

T cells are known to be a vital component of immune-mediated protection against LASV infection [44]. T cells also steer the B cell response and, therefore, a thorough investigation of the T cell response yields insight concerning the mechanisms of both cellular and humoral protection. Despite a strong T cell response, especially with CD4+ populations that are double positive for IFNγ and IL2 (an indication of expanding population), at day 11 after single-dose vaccination there was a low level of IgG antibodies produced at this timepoint. While administration of nAbs in the early stages of LASV infection by passive transfer has shown protection in animal models [45,46], the protection afforded by prior vaccination is thought to be strictly dependent on a T cell response [30,31,35,47,48]. Similarly, multiple vaccine vector platforms that showed high levels of protection in mice, guinea pigs, and NHP have not induced detectable levels of neutralizing Ab (reviewed in Ref 26).

In the 1980s, Clegg and Lloyd [49] expressed Lassa NP from a vaccinia vector and succeeded in protecting guinea pigs, but not primates, from lethal LF disease. Since then, researchers at Porton Down have used a safer vector, MVA, to express LASV NP and protect guinea pigs from LF disease progression [50]. Since they elicited both bAb and a robust cell-mediated immunity to NP in the guinea pig model, it is possible that the MVA-LAS NP could be a standalone vaccine.

GPC is the natural target for nAb responses since it contains epitopes involved in both entry and the endosomal fusion process. GPC, however, is highly glycosylated with 11 N-linked carbohydrate sites on each monomer comprising ~25% of the total mass of the protein, shielding critical residues from Ab access. nAb against GPC have been isolated from the sera of convalescent patients, but these are rare and appear very late in infection [51]. We have consistently elicited excellent functional antibody responses (e.g., bAb, nAb and antibody-dependent cell-mediated cytotoxicity, ADCC) with MVA vaccines that target other viruses such as HIV, Ebola, and Zika [32,33,40,41,50]. A recent publication elicits excellent bAb against an MVA vector expressing LASV NP that has no glycan shield [52]. The low natural bAb against LASV GPC speaks to the effectiveness of the immuno-evasive properties of the protein, including its glycan shield, explaining failures of nAb-based vaccines or therapies using convalescent sera [51]. The combination of the 33 glycans shield, leaving only a few regions vulnerable to antibody binding, and the metastability of the native protein further explain why bAb responses are altogether difficult to elicit by vaccination. Here, we saw robust bAb at d36 (Figure 4d), but that could be attributed to the boost from ML29 virus challenge. Neutralizing antibodies have been isolated from LF survivors as patients were recovering from illness during which the humoral response had time to mature [53]. Recently, by introducing a number of mutations in GPC, this protein could be "locked" in its prefusion state increasing its stability and enabling co-crystallization with human nAb 37.7 H [16]. We are currently exploring whether replacement of the locked GPC structure with native GPC or any other modifications thereof could result in a viable vaccine candidate, demasking the GPC from carbohydrate shields and exposing more epitopes for inducing binding and neutralizing antibodies in vaccinated hosts.

4. Materials and Methods

4.1. Vaccine Construction, Seed Stock Preparation, VLP Formation, and Protein Expression

A recombinant GEO-LM01 was constructed on GeoVax's MVA-VLP platform, utilizing the highly potent yet safe viral vector MVA [54,55]. The vaccine produces two LASV proteins, GPC and Z proteins from Josiah strain LASV lineage IV (GenBank JN650517.1 and JN650518.1). We used a parental MVA that had been harvested in 1974 before the appearance of Bovine Spongiform Encephalopathy /Transmissible Spongiform Encephalopathy (BSE/TSE) and sent in 2001 to Dr. Bernard Moss at NIAID, where it was plaque purified 3 times using certified reagents from sources free of BSE. The pLW76 shuttle vector (Wyatt and Moss, unpublished data) was used to insert the GPC sequences between two essential genes of MVA (I8R and G1L), and LASV Z gene into a restructured and modified deletion III between the A50R and B1R genes. These insertion sites have been identified as supporting high expression and insert stability. All inserted sequences were codon optimized for MVA. Silent mutations were introduced to interrupt homo-polymer sequences (>4G/C and >4A/T), which reduce RNA polymerase errors that possibly lead to frameshifts. The sequences were edited for vaccinia-specific terminators to remove motifs that could lead to premature termination [56]. All vaccine inserts were placed under the modified H5 early/late vaccinia promoter as described previously [57,58]. Vectors, Research Seed Virus (RSV), and Research Stocks (RS) were prepared in a dedicated room at GeoVax, with full traceability and complete documentation of all steps using BSE/TSE-free raw materials and therefore can be directly used for production of cGMP Master Seed Virus (MSV). For production of RSV for animal studies, specific pathogen-free CEF cells were acquired from Charles River Laboratories (cat#10100807), seeded into sterile tissue culture flasks, and infected with GEO-LM01 at MOIs of 0.01. Cells were recovered at 3 days post-infection, disrupted by sonication, and bulk harvest material clarified by low-speed centrifugation. The clarified viral harvest was purified using sucrose cushion ultracentrifugation. The purified viruses were titrated by limiting dilution in DF1 cells, diluted to 1×10^8 $TCID_{50}$/mL in sterile PBS + 7.5% sucrose, dispensed into sterile vials, and stored at −80 °C. Generally, a minimum of 1×10^{10} $TCID_{50}$ of vaccines are produced per mL of harvest material. The VLP formation was evaluated by electron microscopy conducted on thin sections of 48 hour-infected DF-1 cell and was performed at the Emory University Apkarian Integrated Electron Microscopy Core, as previously described [59]. The expression of GPC and Z proteins by MVA was assessed by immunostaining of GEO-LM01 infected DF1 cells that had been fixed in 1:1 methanol:acetone and probed using LASV-specific GPC and Z antibodies (IBT 0307-001, rabbit anti-LASV GP pAb and IBT 0307-002, rabbit anti LASV Z pAb). Plaques were serially diluted (10-fold) from 1:100 to 1:100,000 and stained with anti-GPC or anti-Z monoclonal antibodies, respectively. Similar plaque numbers at each dilution in the GPC and Z wells show that both inserts are retained. The expression of full-length GP1 and GP2 (derived from cleavage of GPC) as well as Z protein, was confirmed by WB analysis conducted on supernatants and lysates of 293T cells 48 hours after infection using standard practices. A pool of human anti-GP1 and -GP2 antibodies (2.4F and 22.5D from Dr. James Robinson, Tulane University, New Orleans, LA) were used as the primary Abs for GP1 and GP2, and a polyclonal rabbit Ab as the primary Ab for Z (IBT Catalog# 0307-002).

4.2. *Mouse Immunogenicity and Efficacy Studies*

4.2.1. **Experiment 1**. Determination of Vaccine Efficacy by Different Routes

Vaccine challenge studies were performed in a mouse model as previously described [24]. Lethality of intracerebrally (IC)-administered ML29 virus was tested in several inbred mouse models and CBA/J mice were the most sensitive to challenge. ML29 is a reassortant virus with its large genome segment from MOPV and its small segment from LASV; subcutaneous administration protects guinea pigs and primates from lethal challenge with LASV [23], but in the absence of vaccination is lethal in this IC challenge model. According to the CDC, ML29 is classified as a BSL3 agent, but not as a Select Agent. In line with University of Maryland Biosafety protocols, all propagation and experiments with high-titer stocks of ML29 virus were performed under BSL3 containment. Day-to-day experiments performed with low-titer stocks were under BSL2 containment. According to biosafety and animal care and use protocols in place, animal studies with low-titer stocks of ML29 virus were performed under ABSL2 containment. The challenge dose was selected based on uniform lethality in unprotected mice as described previously [26]. Immunization doses were based on prior studies testing efficacy of MVA vectored vaccines [38,39].

To determine the best route of immunization, 4–6 week-old CBA/J mice (n = 6) were immunized with 10^7 $TCID_{50}$ of GEO-LM01 by intraperitoneal (IP), intramuscular (IM), or subcutaneous (SC) inoculations. Two groups of mice (n = 6 each) were injected IP with ML29 at 1000 plaque-forming units (PFU) or saline, and served as positive and negative controls, respectively. On day 14, all mice were challenged by IC inoculation with 1000 PFU of ML29 and monitored for weight change, morbidity, and mortality.ML29 titers in the brains of challenged mice were not high enough to be detected by plaque assay. However, ML29 was detectable in a sensitive co-culture assay described in ref [35]. Positive (+) detection was seen in the brains of dying mice, and negative (-) in the brains of surviving mice. Since successfully vaccinated mice survived whereas those given saline or empty vectors succumbed within a week of being challenged, the MVA-Lassa vaccine proved capable of controlling ML29 replication.

4.2.2. **Experiment 2**. Confirmation of Route and Immune Response

A second study to measure immunogenicity and efficacy was initiated in the same model system, in this instance examining only two conditions: immunization with GEO-LM01 by IM inoculation (n = 10) and mock immunization with saline (n = 8). Spleens were harvested from immunized animals (n = 3) and from saline-immunized animals on day 11 after a single administration of the vaccine, and antigen-specific T cell responses were measured by intracellular cytokine staining for IFNγ and IL-2 using LASV GPC immuno-dominant peptides for stimulation. The remaining animals from both groups were challenged on day 14 as in the first experiment. The serum obtained from the 3 animals sacrificed for T cell assays was additionally assayed for the presence of binding antibodies (bAb) against GPC, using ELISA.

4.3. *Splenocyte Isolations and T Cell Assay*

CBA/J mice immunized with saline or once with 10^7 $TCID_{50}$ GEO-LM01 vaccine were sacrificed on day 11 after immunization. Spleens were removed and homogenized through a cell strainer mounted on a 50 mL conical tube in DMEM-10 medium. Cells were centrifuged at 400× g for 5 minutes. Supernatants were aspirated and cells resuspended in 5mL 1× RBC lysis buffer. After 5 minutes at room temperature with occasional shaking, 25 mL HBSS were added to the tube, mixed by inversion, and cells centrifuged at 400× g for 5 minutes. Supernatants were discarded and pellets resuspended in 10mL DMEM-10. Isolated splenocytes were analyzed by ICS following standard protocols. In short, 10^6 splenocytes were stimulated with 0.1µg LASV GP1 (SLYKGVYEL; amino acids 60–68) or GP2 (YLISIFLHL; amino acids 441–480) immuno-dominant epitopes identified within the GPC protein sequence [24–26], or mock stimulated with saline. Incubation proceeded for 6 hours at 37 °C + 5% CO_2; GolgiPlug (BD Biosciences) was added at a concentration of 1.0 µL/mL for the last 4 hours of the incubation. The splenocytes were stained with Live/Dead Fixable Green Dead Cell Stain (ThermoFisher) at room temperature for 20 minutes. The samples were treated with Cytofix/Cytoperm (BD Biosciences) at 4 °C for 20 minutes and were stained with CD3-APC-CY7, CD4-PE-Cy7, CD8-PerCP, IL2-PE, and IFN-γ-Alexa647 (all flow cytometry antibodies from BD Biosciences). Samples were analyzed with a FACSCanto flow cytometer (BD Biosciences) utilizing FACSDiva software. Analysis was performed with FlowJo software. Responses to GP1 and GP2 stimulated cells were added together to represent the total GP stimulated response and then normalized to values from saline stimulated cells. Cytokine responses were scored as a percent of total $CD8^+$ or $CD4^+$ T cells.

4.4. ELISA

Whole blood samples were obtained by retro-orbital bleeding just prior to immunization on days 11–14 post vaccination, and at the termination of experiments. The terminal bleeds shown in Figure 4d were day 36 (22 days following challenge). Sera were obtained by centrifugation of the whole blood samples in serum separator tubes at 3500× g for 5 min. and used to measure bAb in ELISA as described previously [60]. Briefly, flat-bottom 96-well plates were coated overnight at 4 °C with sonication-inactivated ML29 virus, 10^5 PFU/mL in 100 mM bicarbonate buffer, pH 9.6. Plates were washed 4 times with phosphate buffered saline (PBS) + 0.05% Tween-20 (PBST). Next, the plates were blocked with StartingBlock Blocking Buffer (Thermo Fisher Scientific) for 5 minutes at room temperature. Serially-diluted heat-inactivated mouse serum samples were added to wells and incubated for 1 hour at 37 °C. After washing with PBST, goat anti-mouse IgG-HRP (ImmunoReagents) was added to each well and incubated for 1 hour at 37 °C. After a final washing, SureBlue TMB (3,3′, 5, 5′—Tetramethylbenzidine) 1-component substrate solution (KPL) was added to each well, incubated in the dark at room temperature for 10 minutes, and stopped with 1N hydrochloric acid (HCl). Optical density at 450 nm was determined using a Vmax Kinetic ELISA Absorbance Microplate Reader (Molecular Devices). Normalized absorbance values were determined by first subtracting optical density values of blank negative control wells. Endpoint titer was determined by the dilution at which the optical density equaled 0.03.

4.5. Statistical Analyses

Analysis of data was performed using GraphPad Prism (GraphPad Software). Comparisons between groups were performed using a Student's t-test. To test for pairwise differences between groups, an analysis of variance (ANOVA) and Tukey's test of multiple comparisons was performed. Correlations were performed by Spearman rank-correlation tests. A p-value less than 0.05 was considered statistically significant.

4.6. Regulatory Compliance

All methods were carried out in accordance with the relevant guidelines and regulations. All experimental protocols were approved by the University of Maryland School of Medicine Institutional Animal Care and Use Committee (IACUC Protocol # 0217017) and the Institutional Biosafety Committee (approval # IBC-00001495).

5. Conclusions

GEO-LM01 uses GeoVax's MVA-VLP vaccine platform that has been shown to be safe and to induce durable antibody and T cell responses in multiple human clinical trials for GeoVax's prophylactic HIV vaccine. In contrast to other LF vaccines in development that rely on a single glycoprotein antigen, GEO-LM01 includes an additional matrix protein that forms VLPs with the LASV glycoproteins. Upon infection of human cells, the MVA-driven expression of the two proteins leads to the formation of non-infectious VLPs that bear natively-folded glycoproteins on their surface, triggering an effective immune response that is predicted to be more broadly cross-protective than vaccines expressing only one viral antigen [30]. We previously demonstrated that our MVA-VLP-Ebola vaccine conferred full protection after a single dose in non-human primates. This vaccine induced near sterile immunity since no live virus could be detected in the blood of any vaccinated animal post challenge compared to controls (>5$\log_{10}$ $TCID_{50}$ per mL of blood). We are currently evaluating the efficacy of our LF vaccine in guinea pigs and non-human primate models. It remains to be seen whether this vaccine will also be a best-in class vaccine for LF, as shown for the MVA-VLP-Ebola vaccine [61].

Author Contributions: Conceptualization and data curation: M.S., F.G.; Investigation: A.D., C.G.-C., S.M.-M., J.C.Z., H.H., N.M. and R.J.B.; Methodology: M.S., F.G. and A.D.; Project administration: M.H.; Resources: J.C.Z.; Writing—original draft: M.S. and F.G. All authors contributed to reviewing and editing the manuscript.

Funding: This research did not receive any specific grant from funding agencies in the public, commercial, or not-for-profit sectors. Support is acknowledged from the EU Commission Horizon2020 STARBIOS2 grant No. 709517 under Vittorio Colizzi in an effort to promote five key tenets of responsible research and innovation (RRI): public engagement, gender equity, open access, graduate education, and ethical conduct.

Acknowledgments: We thank the Institute of Human Virology staff members Joseph Bryant, Harry Davis, Maurice White, and Sumiko Williams for their excellent contributions to animal husbandry and animal care needs throughout this study. We are indebted to Hong Yi and the Robert P. Apkarian Integrated Electron Microscopy Core of Emory University Medical School for thin section electron microscopy. We are thankful to Erica Saphire from Scripps Institute for providing the molecular structure of the GPC protein and James Robinson from Tulane University for providing antibodies to GP1 and GP2 polypeptides.

Conflicts of Interest: The authors declare competing financial interests: F.G., A.D., M.H. and M.H. are employees of GeoVax, Inc. F.G. and A.D. have pending Patent Application PCT/US2018/043645 Lassa Vaccine Compositions. All other authors have no conflicts or financial disclosures.

References

1. WHO. Epidemic Focus: Lassa fever Weekly Epidemiological Record. Available online: https://www.who.int/wer/2016/wer9121.pdf?ua=1 (accessed on 27 May 2016).
2. Shao, J.; Liang, Y.; Ly, H. Human Hemorrhagic Fever Causing Arenaviruses: Molecular Mechanisms Contributing to Virus Virulence and Disease Pathogenesis. *Pathogens* **2015**, *4*, 283–306. [CrossRef] [PubMed]
3. Leski, T.A.; Stockelman, M.G.; Moses, L.M.; Park, M.; Stenger, D.A.; Ansumana, R.; Bausch, D.G.; Lin, B. Sequence Variability and Geographic Distribution of Lassa Virus, Sierra Leone. *Emerg. Infect. Dis.* **2015**, *21*, 609–618. [CrossRef] [PubMed]
4. McCormick, J.B.; Webb, P.A.; Krebs, J.W.; Johnson, K.M.; Smith, E.S. A Prospective Study of the Epidemiology and Ecology of Lassa Fever. *J. Infect. Dis.* **1987**, *155*, 437–444. [CrossRef] [PubMed]
5. McCormick, J.B. *Lassa Fever, in Emergence and Control of Rodent-Borne Viral Diseases*; Saluzzo, J.F., Dodet, B., Eds.; Elsevier: Amsterdam, The Nertherlands, 1999; pp. 177–195.
6. Richmond, J.K.; Baglole, D.J. Lassa fever: Epidemiology, clinical features, and social consequences. *BMJ* **2003**, *327*, 1271–1275. [CrossRef] [PubMed]
7. Control, N.C.f.D. Disease Situation Reports. 2018. Available online: https://ncdc.gov.ng/diseases/sitreps (accessed on 2 September 2018).
8. Olayemi, A.; Cadar, D.; Magassouba, N.F.; Obadare, A.; Kourouma, F.; Oyeyiola, A.; Fasogbon, S.; Igbokwe, J.; Rieger, T.; Bockholt, S.; et al. New Hosts of The Lassa Virus. *Sci. Rep.* **2016**, *6*, 25280. [CrossRef] [PubMed]
9. Fisher-Hoch, S.P.; Tomori, O.; Nasidi, A.; I Perez-Oronoz, G.; Fakile, Y.; Hutwagner, L.; McCormick, J.B. Review of cases of nosocomial Lassa fever in Nigeria: The high price of poor medical practice. *BMJ* **1995**, *311*, 857–859. [CrossRef] [PubMed]
10. Mylne, A.Q.N.; Pigott, D.M.; Longbottom, J.; Shearer, F.; Duda, K.A.; Messina, J.P.; Weiss, D.J.; Moyes, C.L.; Golding, N.; Hay, S.I. Mapping the zoonotic niche of Lassa fever in Africa. *Trans. R. Soc. Trop. Med. Hyg.* **2015**, *109*, 483–492. [CrossRef] [PubMed]
11. Bowen, M.D.; Rollin, P.E.; Ksiazek, T.G.; Hustad, H.L.; Bausch, D.G.; Demby, A.H.; Bajani, M.D.; Peters, C.J.; Nichol, S.T. Genetic Diversity among Lassa Virus Strains. *J. Virol.* **2000**, *74*, 6992–7004. [CrossRef] [PubMed]
12. Hallam, H.J.; Hallam, S.; Rodriguez, S.E.; Barrett, A.D.T.; Beasley, D.W.C.; Chua, A.; Ksiazek, T.G.; Milligan, G.N.; Sathiyamoorthy, V.; Reece, L.M. Baseline mapping of Lassa fever virology, epidemiology and vaccine research and development. *NPJ Vaccines* **2018**, *3*, 11. [CrossRef]

13. Radoshitzky, S.R.; Bao, Y.; Buchmeier, M.J.; Charrel, R.N.; Clawson, A.N.; Clegg, C.S.; DeRisi, J.L.; Emonet, S.; Gonzalez, J.-P.; Kuhn, J.H.; et al. Past, present, and future of arenavirus taxonomy. *Arch. Virol.* **2015**, *160*, 1851–1874. [CrossRef] [PubMed]
14. Djavani, M.; Lukashevich, I.S.; Sanchez, A.; Nichol, S.T.; Salvato, M.S. Completion of the Lassa fever virus sequence and identification of a RING finger ORF at the L RNA 5′ end. *Virology* **1997**, *235*, 414–418. [CrossRef] [PubMed]
15. Lukashevich, I.S.; Nichol, S.T.; Shapiro, K.; Ravkov, E.; Sanchez, A.; Djavani, M.; Salvato, M.S. The Lassa fever virus L gene: Nucleotide sequence, comparison, and precipitation of a predicted 250 kDa protein with monospecific antiserum. *J. Gen. Virol.* **1997**, *78*, 547–551. [CrossRef] [PubMed]
16. Hastie, K.M.; Zandonatti, M.A.; Kleinfelter, L.M.; Heinrich, M.L.; Rowland, M.M.; Chandran, K.; Branco, L.M.; Robinson, J.E.; Garry, R.F.; Saphire, E.O. Structural basis for antibody-mediated neutralization of Lassa virus. *Science* **2017**, *356*, 923–928. [CrossRef] [PubMed]
17. Lenz, O.; Ter Meulen, J.; Klenk, H.-D.; Seidah, N.G.; Garten, W. The Lassa virus glycoprotein precursor GP-C is proteolytically processed by subtilase SKI-1/S1P. *Proc. Natl. Acad. Sci. USA* **2001**, *98*, 12701–12705. [CrossRef] [PubMed]
18. Ölschläger, S.; Flatz, L. Vaccination Strategies against Highly Pathogenic Arenaviruses: The Next Steps toward Clinical Trials. *PLoS Pathog.* **2013**, *9*, e1003212. [CrossRef] [PubMed]
19. Urata, S.; Yasuda, J. Cis- and cell-type-dependent trans-requirements for Lassa virus-like particle production. *J. Gen. Virol.* **2015**, *96 Pt 7*, 1626–1635. [CrossRef]
20. Safronetz, D.; Mire, C.; Rosenke, K.; Feldmann, F.; Haddock, E.; Geisbert, T.; Feldmann, H. A Recombinant Vesicular Stomatitis Virus-Based Lassa Fever Vaccine Protects Guinea Pigs and Macaques against Challenge with Geographically and Genetically Distinct Lassa Viruses. *PLoS Negl. Trop. Dis.* **2015**, *9*, e0003736. [CrossRef]
21. Verheust, C.; Goossens, M.; Pauwels, K.; Breyer, D. Biosafety aspects of modified vaccinia virus Ankara (MVA)-based vectors used for gene therapy or vaccination. *Vaccine* **2012**, *30*, 2623–2632. [CrossRef]
22. Hastie, K.M.; Zandonatti, M.; Liu, T.; Li, S.; Woods, V.L.; Saphire, E.O. Crystal Structure of the Oligomeric Form of Lassa Virus Matrix Protein Z. *J. Virol.* **2016**, *90*, 4556–4562. [CrossRef]
23. Lukashevich, I.S.; Patterson, J.; Carrion, R.; Moshkoff, D.; Ticer, A.; Zapata, J.; Brasky, K.; Geiger, R.; Hubbard, G.B.; Bryant, J.; et al. A Live Attenuated Vaccine for Lassa Fever Made by Reassortment of Lassa and Mopeia Viruses. *J. Virol.* **2005**, *79*, 13934–13942. [CrossRef]
24. Goicochea, M.A.; Zapata, J.C.; Bryant, J.; Davis, H.; Salvato, M.S.; Lukashevich, I.S. Evaluation of Lassa virus vaccine immunogenicity in a CBA/JML29 mouse model. *Vaccine* **2012**, *30*, 1445–1452. [CrossRef] [PubMed]
25. Botten, J.; Alexander, J.; Pasquetto, V.; Sidney, J.; Barrowman, P.; Ting, J.; Peters, B.; Southwood, S.; Stewart, B.; Rodriguez-Carreno, M.P.; et al. Identification of Protective Lassa Virus Epitopes That Are Restricted by HLA-A2. *J. Virol.* **2006**, *80*, 8351–8361. [CrossRef]
26. Boesen, A.; Sundar, K.; Coico, R. Lassa Fever Virus Peptides Predicted by Computational Analysis Induce Epitope-Specific Cytotoxic-T-Lymphocyte Responses in HLA-A2.1 Transgenic Mice. *Clin. Vaccine Immunol.* **2005**, *12*, 1223–1230. [CrossRef] [PubMed]
27. Kyei, N.N.; Abilba, M.M.; Kwawu, F.K.; Agbenohevi, P.G.; Bonney, J.H.; Agbemaple, T.K.; Nimo-Paintsil, S.C.; Ampofo, W.; Ohene, S.-A.; Nyarko, E.O. Imported Lassa fever: A report of 2 cases in Ghana. *BMC Infect. Dis.* **2015**, *15*, 217. [CrossRef] [PubMed]
28. Mehand, M.S.; Al Shorbaji, F.; Millett, P.; Murgue, B. The WHO R&D Blueprint: 2018 review of emerging infectious diseases requiring urgent research and development efforts. *Antivir. Res.* **2018**, *159*, 63–67. [PubMed]
29. CEPI. News. 2018. Available online: http://cepi.net/news (accessed on 2 September 2018).
30. Zapata, J.C.; Medina-Moreno, S.; Guzmán-Cardozo, C.; Salvato, M.S. Improving the Breadth of the Host's Immune Response to Lassa Virus. *Pathogens* **2018**, *7*, 84. [CrossRef] [PubMed]
31. Ter Meulen, V. Lassa fever: Implications of T-cell immunity for vaccine development. *J. Biotechnol.* **1999**, *73*, 207–212. [CrossRef]
32. Domi, A.; Feldmann, F.; Basu, R.; McCurley, N.; Shifflett, K.; Emanuel, J.; Hellerstein, M.S.; Guirakhoo, F.; Orlandi, C.; Flinko, R.; et al. A Single Dose of Modified Vaccinia Ankara expressing Ebola Virus Like Particles Protects Nonhuman Primates from Lethal Ebola Virus Challenge. *Sci. Rep.* **2018**, *8*, 864. [CrossRef]

33. Brault, A.C.; Domi, A.; McDonald, E.M.; Talmi-Frank, D.; McCurley, N.; Basu, R.; Robinson, H.L.; Hellerstein, M.; Duggal, N.K.; Bowen, R.A.; et al. A Zika Vaccine Targeting NS1 Protein Protects Immunocompetent Adult Mice in a Lethal Challenge Model. *Sci. Rep.* **2017**, *7*, 14769. [CrossRef]
34. Djomand, G.; Quaye, S.; Sullivan, P.S. HIV epidemic among key populations in west Africa. *Curr. Opin. HIV AIDS* **2014**, *9*, 506–513. [CrossRef]
35. Zapata, J.C.; Poonia, B.; Bryant, J.; Davis, H.; Ateh, E.; George, L.; Crasta, O.; Zhang, Y.; Slezak, T.; Jaing, C.; et al. An attenuated Lassa vaccine in SIV-infected rhesus macaques does not persist or cause arenavirus disease but does elicit Lassa virus-specific immunity. *Virol. J.* **2013**, *10*, 52. [CrossRef] [PubMed]
36. Sutter, G.; Moss, B. Nonreplicating vaccinia vector efficiently expresses recombinant genes. *Proc. Natl. Acad. Sci. USA* **1992**, *89*, 10847–10851. [CrossRef] [PubMed]
37. Overton, E.T.; Stapleton, J.; Frank, I.; Hassler, S.; Goepfert, P.A.; Barker, D.; Wagner, E.; Von Krempelhuber, A.; Virgin, G.; Weigl, J.; et al. Safety and Immunogenicity of Modified Vaccinia Ankara-Bavarian Nordic Smallpox Vaccine in Vaccinia-Naive and Experienced Human Immunodeficiency Virus-Infected Individuals: An Open-Label, Controlled Clinical Phase II Trial. *Open Forum Infect. Dis.* **2015**, *2*, ofv040. [CrossRef] [PubMed]
38. Committee for Medicinal Products for Human Use (CHMP). *Assessment Report, IMVANEX, Common Name: Modified Vaccinia Ankara Virus, Procedure No. EMEA/H/C/002596*; Committee for Medicinal Products for Human Use (CHMP), Ed.; European Medicines Agency: London, UK, 2013.
39. Bliss, C.M.; Bowyer, G.; Anagnostou, N.A.; Havelock, T.; Snudden, C.M.; Davies, H.; De Cassan, S.C.; Grobbelaar, A.; Lawrie, A.M.; Venkatraman, N.; et al. Assessment of novel vaccination regimens using viral vectored liver stage malaria vaccines encoding ME-TRAP. *Sci. Rep.* **2018**, *8*, 3390. [CrossRef] [PubMed]
40. Goepfert, P.A.; Elizaga, M.L.; Sato, A.; Qin, L.; Cardinali, M.; Hay, C.M.; Hural, J.; DeRosa, S.C.; Defawe, O.D.; Tomaras, G.D.; et al. Phase 1 Safety and Immunogenicity Testing of DNA and Recombinant Modified Vaccinia Ankara Vaccines Expressing HIV-1 Virus-like Particles. *J. Infect. Dis.* **2011**, *203*, 610–619. [CrossRef] [PubMed]
41. Goepfert, P.A.; Elizaga, M.L.; Seaton, K.; Tomaras, G.D.; Montefiori, D.C.; Sato, A.; Hural, J.; DeRosa, S.C.; Kalams, S.A.; McElrath, M.J.; et al. Specificity and 6-Month Durability of Immune Responses Induced by DNA and Recombinant Modified Vaccinia Ankara Vaccines Expressing HIV-1 Virus-Like Particles. *J. Infect. Dis.* **2014**, *210*, 99–110. [CrossRef] [PubMed]
42. Thompson, M.; Heath, S.L.; Sweeton, B.; Williams, K.; Cunningham, P.; Keele, B.F.; Sen, S.; Palmer, B.E.; Chomont, N.; Xu, Y.; et al. DNA/MVA Vaccination of HIV-1 Infected Participants with Viral Suppression on Antiretroviral Therapy, followed by Treatment Interruption: Elicitation of Immune Responses without Control of Re-Emergent Virus. *PLoS ONE* **2016**, *11*, 0163164. [CrossRef]
43. Maciel, M.M., Jr.; Cruz, F.D.S.P.; Cordeiro, M.T.; da Motta, M.A.; de Melo Cassemiro, K.M.S.; Maia, R.D.C.C.; de Figueiredo, R.C.B.Q.; Galler, R.; da Silva Freire, M.; August, J.T.; et al. A DNA Vaccine against Yellow Fever Virus: Development and Evaluation. *PLoS Negl. Trop. Dis.* **2015**, *9*, e0003693. [CrossRef]
44. Perdomo-Celis, F.; Salvato, M.S.; Medina-Moreno, S.; Zapata, J.C. T-Cell Response to Viral Hemorrhagic Fevers. *Vaccines* **2019**, *7*, 11. [CrossRef]
45. Cross, R.W.; Mire, C.E.; Branco, L.M.; Geisbert, J.B.; Rowland, M.M.; Heinrich, M.L.; Goba, A.; Momoh, M.; Grant, D.S.; Fullah, M.; et al. Treatment of Lassa virus infection in outbred guinea pigs with first-in-class human monoclonal antibodies. *Antivir. Res.* **2016**, *133*, 218–222. [CrossRef]
46. Mire, C.E.; Cross, R.W.; Geisbert, J.B.; Borisevich, V.; Agans, K.N.; Deer, D.J.; Heinrich, M.L.; Rowland, M.M.; Goba, A.; Momoh, M.; et al. Human-monoclonal-antibody therapy protects nonhuman primates against advanced Lassa fever. *Nat. Med.* **2017**, *23*, 1146–1149. [CrossRef] [PubMed]
47. Lukashevich, I.S.; Carrion, R.; Salvato, M.S.; Mansfield, K.; Brasky, K.; Zapata, J.; Cairo, C.; Goicochea, M.; Hoosien, G.E.; Ticer, A.; et al. Safety, immunogenicity, and efficacy of the ML29 reassortant vaccine for Lassa fever in small non-human primates. *Vaccine* **2008**, *26*, 5246–5254. [CrossRef] [PubMed]
48. Kiley, M. Protection of Rhesus Monkeys from Lassa Virus by Immunisation With Closely Related Arenavirus. *Lancet* **1979**, *314*, 738. [CrossRef]
49. Clegg, J.; Lloyd, G. Vaccinia Recombinant Expressing Lassa-Virus Internal Nucleocapsid Protein Protects Guinea pigs against Lassa Fever. *Lancet* **1987**, *330*, 186–188. [CrossRef]
50. McCurley, N.P.; Domi, A.; Basu, R.; Saunders, K.O.; Labranche, C.C.; Montefiori, D.C.; Haynes, B.F.; Robinson, H.L. HIV transmitted/founder vaccines elicit autologous tier 2 neutralizing antibodies for the CD4 binding site. *PLoS ONE* **2017**, *12*, e0177863. [CrossRef] [PubMed]

51. Sommerstein, R.; Flatz, L.; Remy, M.M.; Malinge, P.; Magistrelli, G.; Fischer, N.; Sahin, M.; Bergthaler, A.; Igonet, S.; Ter Meulen, J.; et al. Arenavirus Glycan Shield Promotes Neutralizing Antibody Evasion and Protracted Infection. *PLoS Pathog.* **2015**, *11*, e1005276. [CrossRef] [PubMed]
52. Kennedy, E.; Dowall, S.; Salguero, F.; Yeates, P.; Aram, M.; Hewson, R. A vaccine based on recombinant modified Vaccinia Ankara containing the nucleoprotein from Lassa virus protects against disease progression in a guinea pig model. *Vaccine* **2019**, *37*, 5404–5413. [CrossRef] [PubMed]
53. Robinson, J.E.; Hastie, K.M.; Cross, R.W.; Yenni, R.E.; Elliott, D.H.; Rouelle, J.A.; Kannadka, C.B.; Smira, A.A.; Garry, C.E.; Bradley, B.T.; et al. Most neutralizing human monoclonal antibodies target novel epitopes requiring both Lassa virus glycoprotein subunits. *Nat. Commun.* **2016**, *7*, 11544. [CrossRef]
54. Altenburg, A.F.; Kreijtz, J.H.C.M.; De Vries, R.D.; Song, F.; Fux, R.; Rimmelzwaan, G.F.; Sutter, G.; Volz, A. Modified Vaccinia Virus Ankara (MVA) as Production Platform for Vaccines against Influenza and Other Viral Respiratory Diseases. *Viruses* **2014**, *6*, 2735–2761. [CrossRef]
55. Moss, B.; Carroll, M.W.; Wyatt, L.S.; Bennink, J.R.; Hirsch, V.M.; Goldstein, S.; Elkins, W.R.; Fuerst, T.R.; Lifson, J.D.; Piatak, M.; et al. Host Range Restricted, Non-Replicating Vaccinia Virus Vectors as Vaccine Candidates. *Results Probl. Cell Differ.* **1996**, *397*, 7–13.
56. Wyatt, L.S.; Earl, P.L.; Vogt, J.; Eller, L.A.; Chandran, D.; Liu, J.; Robinson, H.L.; Moss, B. Correlation of immunogenicities and in vitro expression levels of recombinant modified vaccinia virus Ankara HIV vaccines. *Vaccine* **2008**, *26*, 486–493. [CrossRef] [PubMed]
57. Wyatt, L.S.; Earl, P.L.; Xiao, W.; Americo, J.L.; Cotter, C.A.; Vogt, J.; Moss, B. Elucidating and Minimizing the Loss by Recombinant Vaccinia Virus of Human Immunodeficiency Virus Gene Expression Resulting from Spontaneous Mutations and Positive Selection. *J. Virol.* **2009**, *83*, 7176–7184. [CrossRef] [PubMed]
58. Earl, P.L.; Cotter, C.; Moss, B.; VanCott, T.; Currier, J.; Eller, L.A.; McCutchan, F.; Birx, D.L.; Michael, N.L.; Marovich, M.A.; et al. Design and evaluation of multi-gene, multi-clade HIV-1 MVA vaccines. *Vaccine* **2009**, *27*, 5885–5895. [CrossRef] [PubMed]
59. Hellerstein, M.; Xu, Y.; Marino, T.; Lu, S.; Yi, H.; Wright, E.R.; Robinson, H.L. Co-expression of HIV-1 virus-like particles and granulocyte-macrophage colony stimulating factor by GEO-D03 DNA vaccine. *Hum. Vaccines Immunother.* **2012**, *8*, 1654–1658. [CrossRef] [PubMed]
60. Salvato, M.S.; Lukashevich, I.S.; Medina-Moreno, S.; Zapata, J.C. *Diagnostics for Lassa Fever: Detecting Host Antibody Responses, in Hemorrhagic Fever Viruses: Methods and Protocols*; Humana Press: New York, NY, USA, 2018.
61. Lázaro-Frías, A.; Gomez-Medina, S.; Sánchez-Sampedro, L.; Ljungberg, K.; Ustav, M.; Liljeström, P.; Muñoz-Fontela, C.; Esteban, M.; García-Arriaza, J. Distinct Immunogenicity and Efficacy of Poxvirus-Based Vaccine Candidates against Ebola Virus Expressing GP and VP40 Proteins. *J. Virol.* **2018**, *92*, e00363–e00418. [CrossRef]